THE POLITICAL ECONOMY OF STIGMA

THE POLITICAL ECONOMY OF STIGMA

HIV, MEMOIR, MEDICINE, AND CRIP POSITIONALITIES

Ally Day

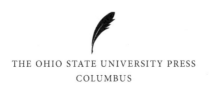

THE OHIO STATE UNIVERSITY PRESS

COLUMBUS

Library of Congress Cataloging-in-Publication Data can be found online at http://catalog.
loc.gov.

Cover design by Angela Moody
Text composition by Stuart Rodriguez
Type set in Minion Pro

♾ The paper used in this publication meets the minimum requirements of the American
National Standard for Information Sciences—Permanence of Paper for Printed Library
Materials. ANSI Z39.48-1992.

For R. E. D.
for whom a book about books seems most appropriate

CONTENTS

ACKNOWLEDGMENTS

I was in the first day of Professor Wendy Hesford's graduate class at OSU when she implored us to read the acknowledgments of our assigned monographs. This was a class about autobiographic subjectivity, and she asked us to consider these often overlooked pages as forms of autobiography, a way to understand the intellectual and personal history of our theorists. A decade and a half later, remembering Professor Hesford's lesson, I feel more intimidated than ever to write these acknowledgments.

I have many people and institutions to thank. I want to begin by thanking the research participants who engaged with me for months and put their trust in this project; without them, there is no book. Special thanks to The Ohio State University Press for taking a chance on this project, particularly Taralee Cyphers and all the anonymous peer reviewers who have strengthened this work. I also want to thank the University of Toledo Office of Research and Sponsored Programs, The Ohio State University's Elizabeth D. Gee Research Grant for Women's Gender and Sexuality Studies, and the Arts and Humanities Graduate Research Grant for funding various components of this research.

I am one of the lucky ones who landed a dream job; I am deeply grateful to my colleagues in the University of Toledo Disability Studies Program, past and present, including Kim Nielsen (the best mentor a feminist scholar could ask for), Liat Ben Moshe (oh, the trouble we can cause), Dean Adams, Jim Ferris, Josh Kupetz, Alison Kopit, and Becca Monteleone. Building a program with this group has been tremendously fun, and I know because of the talent I engage with every day that I am a deeper thinker and more compassionate person than I was ten years ago. I am also grateful to many in the larger DST community who shared meals, responded to anxious emails, and danced. Particular thanks to Sami Schalk, Jess Waggoner, Aimi Hamraie, Sandi Yi, Kate Caldwell, Margaret Fink, Leslie Frye, Aly Patsavas, Jina Kim, Akemi Nishida, Angela Carter, Olivia Banner, Stacy Simplican Clifford, Alison Kafer, Margaret Price, Julie Elman, Stephanie Kerschbaum, Susan Burch, Eli Clare, Leah Laksmi Piepzna-Samarasinha, Mike Rembis, and Jay Dolmage.

I also continue to be encouraged and supported by a large network of UT colleagues, including Linda Curtis, Sharon Barnes, Asma Abdel Halim, Jeanne Kusina, Melissa Baltus, Tom Zych, Kim McBride, Chelsea Griffis, Kristen Geaman, Holly Hey (and Lee!), Joey Gamble, and Kasumi Yamazaki. Additional thanks to my vagina writing group: Renee Heberle, Shelley Cavalieri, Beth Currans, Liat Ben Moshe, and Mysoon Rizk. And special thanks to all of my students, past and present, who push me every. single. day.

Before coming to UT, I was surrounded by incredible people at The Ohio State University, including my comrades Deema Kaedbey, Brena Tai, Andrea Gulino, Lindsey Bernhagen, Lois Kwa, Meredith Lee, and Judy Rodriguez— you guys are a lifeline. Additional thanks to the Women's Gender and Sexuality Studies Department, including Wendy Smooth, Shannon Winnubst, Rebecca Wanzo, Kimberly Springer, Guisela Latorre, Judy Wu, Cricket Keating, Lynn Itagaki, Anne Mitchell, Varsha Chitnis, Nikki Frances, Anindita Sengupta, and Debanuj DasGupta. Unending gratitude to Brenda Brueggemann for introducing me to the field of disability studies and for being nothing but a cheerleader from day one.

If there is one academic program that truly and deeply affected me, it is the Simmons College Gender and Cultural Studies Program, whose professors are world-class feminists, researchers, and pedagogues: unending gratitude to Becky Thompson, Jyoti Puri, Jo Trigilio, Sarah Leonard, and Theresa Perry. In addition to the professors, the comrade scholars who joined me in this program are truly remarkable, producing incredible work in and outside of academic communities and continuing to be some of the best friends one can ask for. Many thanks to my Simmons Siblings: Candace Cheatham (girl—that first Foucault reading . . .), Gwen Warman, Shana Russell, Brenda Sanya, Jess Guerrero, and Meiver de la Cruz. And of course, my best friend and partner, Catherine Harrington.

I would have never made it to Simmons without the lifesaving community (quite literally) of UMaine Farmington. Special and deep gratitude for two incredible mentors and professors, Jim Melcher and Gretchen Legler, and the best roommates and comrades a girl could ask for: Prema Long, Ashley Nadeau, Jim Doucette, PJ Oxman, and Say Carnahan. And my Maine thank-yous would not be nearly complete without recognizing the incredible mentors Claire Holman and Anita Charles, for whom I did some of my first autobiographical writing.

Many thanks to the communities who have supported me during the writing and revising of this book, including Laila Hanson's "meetup," Broadmead Quakers, Yogaja and Hot Room yoga studios, and the GCCF "noon" crew. I have been well fed by Toledo restaurants offering gf comfort food, including Sidon, Zaza, Pizza Cat, Carlos Poco Loco, and Sip Coffee. I am grateful to continue to hone my poker skills with "the crew" (The Silver Fox, Kim, Melissa, and Tom) and my media habits with my Rogers Park comrades (Reem, Annie, Pam, Linde, Hannah—additional thanks to Reem, Annie, and Linde, who have read and helped me improve portions of my work).

And of course, I would not be here without my family. Deep thanks for my grandparents Bob, Anna, Shirley, and Diz, as well as for my Uncle David and Aunt Linda—your influence and love have been boundless. Thanks to my parents and sisters for keeping me grounded—arguments, celebrations, and all. I will always be the obnoxious youngest sibling and troublemaker, and I thank you for giving me that place of honor. Thanks to all my nieces and nephews (Henry, CeCe, Sammy, Anders, Serena, Miles, Dylan) for being unendingly hilarious. And to my Quinsig girls (Liri, Jess, Jen, Cara, Lea) for the roller-skating routines and long walks to school. And to my chosen family, Gretchen and Ruth (my aunties) Meiver, Ashley, Prema, and Matt—there are not enough words.

There is one person who has been there day in and day out for more than twelve years. Every day I have renewed love for my partner, Cat, whose humor, courage, wicked smarts, and love make our home a place of daily adventure and respite. You make this all possible. And while this may sound trite, I would be remiss if I did not thank the various fur family who warmed my lap over the course of writing this book: Bob, Diz, Scruffy, Abby, Oscar Wilde, and Burger. Thanks for helping to keep the heating bill down.

Portions of the analysis in chapter 2 were published in early versions in "Postfeminist Motherhood? Reading a Differential Deployment of Identity in American Women's HIV Narrative," in *Disabling Domesticity*, edited by Michael Rembis (Palgrave Macmillan, 2016), pp. 309–33; and "Embodied Triumph and Political Mobilization: Reading Marvelyn Brown's *The Naked Truth: Young, Beautiful and (HIV) Positive*," in *a/b: Journal of Autobiography* vol. 28, no.1, 2013, pp. 112–25; both are reprinted with permission. Additional scenes and analysis from the introduction and chapter 3 appear in "Doing Disability

Autobiography as Feminist Disability Praxis," in *Research Methodologies for Auto/biography Studies,* edited by Kate Douglas and Ashley Barnwell (Routledge, 2019), pp. 186–92, and "Resisting Disability, Claiming HIV: Introducing the Ability Contract and Conceptualizations of Liberal Citizenship," in *The Canadian Journal of Disability Studies* vol. 3, no. 3, 2014, pp. 104–21. Both are reprinted with permission.

INTRODUCTION

Disability, HIV, and the Political Economy of Stigma

I have been meeting and reading with a group of women living with HIV for months. We've been spending late afternoons once a week together, talking about HIV memoir. This week we are discussing Regan Hoffman's mass-market memoir *I've Got Something to Tell You*, which recounts the experience of contracting HIV from the perspective of a White, well-educated, and wealthy Gen X woman on the East Coast. I ask, in what has become our usual ritual, whether anyone wants to begin by giving us a brief summary of what they have read so far. One of the group participants leans back in her chair, holds the book out over the table as she stretches her legs, and pronounces, "To be honest, I couldn't get past the image of her and her damn horse!" The other members erupt in laughter, nodding in agreement in their distaste for the book cover, which features a photograph of a White woman with cascading blonde hair obscuring her face, seated on a brown horse and surrounded by pasture. They are responding as women living with HIV, Black and White, working-class, neither East Coast nor West Coast but rust-belt dwellers.

A few years later, I am hosting another reading group, this time with AIDS service workers in another rust-belt city. We are also discussing Hoffman's memoir, but for this group, the book would be an overwhelming favorite. One

---

1. All research participants in my reading group research are given pseudonyms to protect their anonymity.

of my participants, a White gay man with a graduate degree, tells the group, "This book actually made me cry. It was like 'oh.' It's like that doesn't usually happen with books with me." Around the table, I notice others nodding (9/8/2015). The book this group disliked the most was the oldest HIV memoir we read in both groups, *AIDS Memoir: Journal of an HIV-Positive Mother,* written by Catherine Wyatt-Morley, a religious African American woman in the Deep South in the mid-1990s. The AIDS service workers group understood Wyatt-Morley as "historical" and "no longer relevant," perhaps also related to the memoir's cover, which features three family photos of Wyatt-Morley with her children, easy to date with hair and fashion as the early 1990s. In contrast, the group composed of women living with HIV felt a distinct connection to the writing of Catherine Wyatt-Morley and found her book to be the most relatable one they read during our time together. Unlike with other authors, this group referred to Wyatt-Morley by her first name, Catherine, and consistently circled back to her story as we read other books. Most notably, it was while discussing Wyatt-Morley's book that they shared the most about their own experience with work, medical care, and the process of their own complicated HIV disclosures.

What explains this discrepancy in reader reception? How can the group of AIDS service workers have such a different perspective from the group of women living with HIV? In what follows, I recount and analyze my experience with these two reading groups—that is, women living with HIV and AIDS service workers—in order to address the divergent impact of narrative on medicine and care. *The Political Economy of Stigma* provides a methodological innovation: a reading group praxis for creating theory through narrative and medicine that is collaborative, critical, and creative. It also provides a theoretical apparatus for reading and interpreting disability and illness narrative within a neoliberal medical economy; I call this apparatus the *political economy of stigma*. I define the political economy of stigma as the formal and informal circulation of personal illness and disability narrative that benefits some while hindering others. On the one hand, the political economy of stigma works to decrease access to appropriate medical care for those with chronic, unpredictable conditions by producing narratives of personal illness that frame one's relationship to structural inequality as a result of personal failure. On the other hand, the political economy of stigma rewards those who procure such narratives, such as medical practitioners, and circulate these narratives for public consumption, either in publications or in professional education settings. While not all narratives of illness and disability circulate within the political economy of stigma (for instance, can a doctor living with HIV treating patients living with HIV be neatly encompassed in the binary positionalities of the political economy of stigma? How about a doctor disabled by Parkinson's treating HIV patients?), the political economy of stigma as an apparatus for analysis can help us understand why some memoirs are more popular than others, why some patient case studies are written about by doctors, and why mainstream reader interpretation remains entrenched in stigmatizing tropes, such as pity and triumph, elaborated on frequently by disability life-writing theorists.

My research works with people living with HIV, and affected by HIV, because, as Susan Sontag most famously theorized, HIV is *the* stigmatizing condition of our time. While Sontag is writing about HIV stigma forty years ago, the stigma for those living with and affected by HIV shifts and evolves but does not evaporate. At the time of writing this introduction, African Americans make up half of those living with HIV; HIV-related illness is still the third leading cause of death among Black women ages twenty-five to forty-four and Black men ages thirty-five to forty-four (Centers for Disease Control n.d.). According to the first US-based HIV Stigma Index Study, 73 percent of people living with HIV experience discrimination as a result of their serostatus, and 20 percent report explicit discrimination in housing, health care, or insurance coverage (People Living with HIV Stigma Index n.d.). This project directly addresses the experience of disability oppression and stigma through an intersectional analysis of gender, race, class, and citizenship—this at a time when the forty-fifth president of the US dismantled the President's Advisory Council on AIDS and proposed forty million dollars in budget cuts to the CDC for HIV-related research.[2] *The Political Economy of Stigma* proposes one way to understand this shapeshifter of stigma that is particular to the early twenty-first century and neoliberal governmentality. Moreover, in what follows, I show how that neoliberal governmentality is alive and well within the production of memoir and the growing academic/professional fields of the

---

2. In December 2017 the forty-fifth US president was quoted as saying earlier that year that Haitian immigrants "all have AIDS"; this is in the context of justifying increasingly restrictive immigration from countries in Africa and Central and South America, what President Trump in the same conversation called "shithole countries." While the White House refutes this explicit language, what remains unrefuted is the stigma of HIV itself. Indeed, very little media coverage attempted to unpack why "AIDS" would be a reason to restrict immigration, despite the fact that in October 2009 President Obama lifted the twenty-two-year ban on HIV-positive immigrants, telling reporters, "If we want to be a global leader in combating H.I.V./AIDS, we need to act like it. Now, we talk about reducing the stigma of this disease, yet we've treated a visitor living with it as a threat." By the end of December 2017 (ironically the month that begins with World's AIDS Day, a designation made in 1988), Trump had fired all members of the Presidential Advisory Council on HIV/AIDS. In February 2018 the Trump administration proposed significant budget cuts in HIV/AIDS prevention and treatment, including forty million dollars to the CDC.

medical humanities and how it is against this backdrop that the political economy of stigma operates.

The political economy of stigma affirms how theorist Ross Chambers understands that HIV writing "may be accommodationist as well as socially transformative in intention or effect" (21).[3] In other words, published memoirs, as well as the formal and informal spoken-narrative accounts of HIV, can at times reinforce dangerous tropes of personal responsibility or shame and, at other times, resist these same understandings. I argue that narratives of HIV are deployed with attention to power that shapes the narrative strategy of the teller; witnesses are not always aware of this negotiation, missing the teller's intention.

We can understand this disconnect between a narrator's intention and the reader-witness's interpretation by examining the growing popularity of narrative medicine. Narrative medicine, a branch of the medical humanities housed at Columbia University, educates medical providers in narrative interpretation in order to address some of the problems of increasingly short doctor–patient visits and the larger problems of the depersonalized and bureaucratic medical system. This project looks closely at the pedagogical approaches of narrative medicine, and its adaptation in settings outside of Columbia University; doing so, I find that narrative medicine practitioners risk exploiting the privacy of patients while being rewarded within a neoliberal medical system for obtaining another specialization. My critique of narrative medicine as a pedagogical and medical practice is that, like narrative itself, it is messy, imperfect, and contradictory. It also can dangerously reinforce systems of medical and social injustice.

The political economy of stigma is plagued by contradictions in subjectivity—a kind of narrative messiness—because it is a product of neoliberalism. Indeed, I argue that through the mediation of author–reader relationships, the political economy of stigma is created. This extends Robert McRuer's analysis of the complexity of stigmatization within neoliberalism (2018). My analysis contributes to an understanding that under neoliberalism, difference itself can be celebrated and then contained by funneling it into the market (17–19). The political economy of stigma that I propose is one mechanism through which we can understand *crip theory*, a term and field that, in Carrie Sandahl's (2003) formulation, is meant to be expansive and open-ended and, in Alison Kafer's

---

3. Ross Chambers points to a key problem in the work of Arthur Frank in *The Wounded Storyteller*, which too often understands narrative as unitary. Like Chambers, the political economy of stigma proposes that we understand narrative not as "direct, straight-forward and unproblematic" (18) but as a negotiated practice "exclusively determined by the subjective nature of the (whether damaged or whole) the storyteller" (19).

(2003) understanding, is meant to disrupt the binaries of social and medical models. *Crip,* as a term, is always attentive to power dynamics as it disrupts binaries; here, I do not argue that there is a correct interpretation of HIV memoir or a binary relationship of the "good" narrative producer and the "bad" medical practitioner. Crip theory provides me the theoretical tools to highlight how power operates in the lives of those with disability and chronic illness. One way that power operates is to ask us to divide subjectivities into simple binaries: disabled/able-bodied, doctor/patient, teller/witness. Power, as Eli Clare reminds us, asks us to diagnose, to delineate concrete boundaries around conditions and symptoms (2017). Crip theory asks us to resist these boundaries, to recognize diagnosis as one operation of power. I use *crip* in my title to highlight how subjectivities themselves reflect a mobile relationship to power and deeply affect our own interpretations of narrative. Ultimately, this project is deeply invested in the political possibilities of memoir, medicine, and the relationship between the two that moves us beyond diagnosis and toward a more just practice of storytelling about disability and illness.

How do we tell stories about illness and disability? How do we receive each other's stories about illness and disability? How do these stories circulate as a practice of belonging? How we answer these questions can help us understand the role that storytelling plays in how we access medical resources. If our story of illness is readily understandable by a medical practitioner, perhaps because our story displays symptoms of diabetes and because we are recognized as a member of a population within which this diagnosis is prominent, then that medical practitioner can enter into their charts the correct insurance billing code and begin to prescribe treatments. If our condition is not readily identifiable, for instance, those who understand themselves as having chronic Lyme disease,[4] then treatment becomes less accessible—there is no code to cover insurance billing, there is no recommended treatment by the American Medical Association. How we tell the stories of our symptoms has a direct implication for our treatment; what we withhold is often a carefully calculated negotiation of medical expectation and our own pursuits of privacy.

HIV Crip Theory and Feminist Disability Studies

In the past fifteen years, as we have moved to more quantifiable, population-based standards for health care with the rise of evidence-based medicine,

---

4. For more on the debate between mainstream physicians and "Lyme-literate" physicians, see Dumes.

there has been a corresponding interest in training medical practitioners to be skilled storytellers and listeners. One of the most prominent places where we see this interest is in the growth of narrative medicine, a subfield of the medical humanities founded and housed at Columbia University. *The Political Economy of Stigma* explores these questions about medical storytelling within narrative medicine because narrative medicine provides us a case study for how interest in narrative can be diverted from its transformative potential and used to uphold the status quo of an inequitable and broken medical system. Broadly, I ask, what would an approach to narrative and medicine look like if it used a feminist disability studies lens and method? How might we understand and use narrative within medicine if we were held accountable to the political transformation of medicine?

In the last quarter of the twentieth century, there was movement toward the transformation of medicine with the activism of the AIDS crisis. As Celeste Watkins-Hayes notes, this activism built a "gold standard" of care because it created a broad social net to address the social dimensions of client/patient lives, not simply medical diagnosis (202–3). However, with the advance and promotion of drugs that can allow someone living with the virus to remain undetectable, and thus much less likely to spread the virus because of the suppression of their viral load, there is a move to dismantle this safety net in favor of a "test-and-treat revolution" (178–203). Watkins-Hayes, in collecting the life stories of women living with HIV in the greater Chicago area, reminds us of the importance of narrative in our ongoing pursuit of medical transformation: "I would point to the significance of storytelling in the AIDS response. Its centrality cannot be overstated as a defining characteristic of the HIV safety net" (245). Because of our current precarious moment in relation to the HIV safety net, and its transformative effects in the lives of those living with or affected by HIV, and that safety net's relationship to storytelling, *The Political Economy of Stigma* centers the experience of HIV. Both AIDS service providers and women living with HIV provide valuable insight into the circulation of narrative within medicine, giving us more tools for understanding the pros and cons of narrative medicine.

While scholarly monographs and collections addressing the HIV crisis in the US have proliferated since the mid-1990s, little attention has been given to how women memoirists living with HIV have contributed to our understandings of disability, chronic illness, and citizenship. These memoirs challenge dominant understandings of HIV as a White homosexual[5] male experience;

---

5. I use *homosexual* here because much of the early first-person accounts of HIV are written by people who identify as homosexual men. See, for example, the work of Paul Monette.

this is where I begin with my exploration of HIV subjectivity and stigma. Others have conceptualized how HIV has been central to the development of queer theory. As such, these memoirs written by women living with HIV aim to reshape both HIV activism and the work of AIDS service organizations, as well as academic epistemologies of the fast-growing field of crip theory, which addresses the intersection of disability studies and queer theory. Robert McRuer identifies crip theory as a way to account for compulsory able-bodied-ness, analogous to compulsory heterosexuality, and the ways in which identities once considered radical become co-opted into the transnational flow of neoliberal markets (16–18). My project is concerned with crip theory precisely because it interrogates the tangle of disability, sexuality, and the production of identification through HIV life writing; indeed, queer theory, crip theory, and HIV have a complicated entanglement to which this project pays homage.[6]

This project has also been influenced by those disability theorists who have engaged with the work of Michel Foucault. As Shelley Tremain writes, the field of disability studies has been deepened by scholars' responding to Foucault's call "to interrogate what has been regarded as natural, inevitable, ethical and liberating through an analysis of widely endorsed practices and ideas surrounding disability," including those in medical fields (11). If we understand government, as Foucault calls us to, as any "activity that aims to shape, guide or affect the conduct of some person or persons" (16), then we can understand the political economy of stigma, and its operation through the memoir industry, as a form of governmentality. At the foundation of this project is the assumption that life writing, and the memoir industry in particular, circulates as a mechanism to reinforce ideals of good citizenship—whose stories become legible is determined by understandings of citizenship and belonging.

---

6. One inaugural article in the field of queer theory is Leo Bersani's "Is the Rectum the Grave?" Written in the midst of the HIV crisis of the late 1980s, Bersani's piece highlights how AIDS represents not just a medical crisis but a representational crisis (198). He argues, using Stuart Hall, that HIV coverage is geared toward a low-risk, heterosexual nuclear family; the high-risk groups remain invisible as an audience (203). Bersani proposes, in light of the stereotypes of homosexuality, that we understand anal penetration not as a place where one abdicates power but as a place where masculine subjectivity itself is buried (211, 221–22). In responding to White anti-penetration feminists Andrea Dworkin and Katherine MacKinnon, Bersani stakes a claim not to rehabilitate sexual acts of penetration but to value sex for the very shattering of self that it produces (222). Queer theory emerges to deconstruct ideologies of the self and to unveil particular understandings of performativity from Judith Butler's *Gender Trouble*; crip and disability theorists who have taken up these ideas include Ellen Samuels (2003), Alison Kafer (2003), Sami Schalk (2013), Robert McRuer (2006), and others. Lisa Diedrich's 2016 monograph explicitly lays out provocative connections between the development of queer theory and the experience of HIV.

I explore stigma, narrative, and medicine through crip theory and the overlapping lens of feminist disability studies. Feminist disability studies is a theoretical field that combines feminist methodology and feminist interpretation with disability studies; this includes paying sharp attention to power and intersectional oppression and developing theoretical tools that can lead to social and material change (Hawkesworth 3–11, 17–53). While several feminist texts inspired this project, two serve as a foundation that are not frequently addressed in the context of disability studies, Joan Scott's "Evidence of Experience" and Gayatri Spivak's "Can the Subaltern Speak?" Scott argues that what is important in our interpretation of history and narrative is understanding how particular identities become available (790–97). In this project, I am interested not just in how one identifies as disabled/HIV-positive/Black/queer but also how particular kinds of identity become available at particular moments of political negotiation—how one identifies is always already a negotiation of power. Scott concludes that experience is "not the origin of our explanation, but that which we want to explain" (797). Experience is important because it is simultaneously already an interpretation and something that needs to be interpreted (797). Foundational to this project is the understanding that experience is not self-evident; experience is a representation of particular power relations. When Gayatri Spivak asks us whether the subaltern can speak, she is similarly looking to power relations in her analysis of experience. For Spivak, the subaltern can and does speak but is frequently unheard because of essentializing practices of colonialism, classism, and sexism (38–44, 1988). I propose that by beginning a feminist disability studies project with the foundation of Scott and Spivak, I am broadening a field that has been criticized as too White- and too Western-centric (disability studies) and a field that has been too ableist (feminist studies) in order to conceptualize a relationship between stigma, medicine, and narrative; I do so alongside women living with HIV who are poor, working-class, Brown, White, and marginalized.

As stated earlier, I propose a contribution to theory about stigma through my concept of the political economy of stigma, a concept that accounts for the circulation and appropriation of personal narrative within a neoliberal medical system that increasingly conceptualizes medical intervention as a responsibility of individuals. Here, those whose narratives adhere to an individualizing ethos of personal responsibility are received by medical practitioners through empathetic relationships and rewarded with efficient and appropriate medical care; those whose narratives reflect complex systems of oppression are stigmatized, their narratives circulated as examples of noncompliance and personal failures.[7] The political economy of stigma, as an analytical apparatus, accounts for the seemingly infinite circulation of stigma.

Stigma[8] must be understood within a neoliberal political context as a product that circulates to reinforce the citizen-consumer's feeling of belonging.[9] In making this argument, I draw on several disability studies scholars. For example, Tanya Titchkovsky argues that stigma isn't so much about "two piles of people," one the stigmatizer and one the stigmatized, but about the place "between attribute and stereotype." With HIV-related illness as its context, the political economy of stigma extends Titchkovsky's analysis by offering a case study for how stigma can be what she calls a "social regulation of belonging and participation." The political economy of stigma mediates relationships between authors and readers textually and paratextually in disabil-

---

7. At the foundation of my scholarship here are feminist activist-scholars like Cindy Patton and her 2005 book *Last Served? Gendering the HIV Pandemic* and Evelynn Hammonds's body of research, including the 1997 article "Seeing AIDS: Race, Gender and Representation." Many scholars, notably Cathy Cohen and Michele Berger, have written excellent works about HIV and gender discrimination in the recognition of the virus in communities of color, in the allocation of resources for care and research, and in the way our understanding of the virus has been shaped by gendered, racialized, colonized "common sense." More recently, scholars like Deborah Gould and Priscilla Wald have written comprehensive histories of the rhetoric of the AIDS epidemic (Wald) and the affective work of activist groups such as ACT UP (Gould) that have generated important insights into how we understand disease as part of a larger political landscape. Any discussion of HIV and stigma is necessarily indebted to the theoretical formulations of Susan Sontag, who writes of AIDS stigma as eclipsing cancer (99–104); AIDS's "capacity to create a spoiled identity" (104), understood as both an invasion (like cancer) and a pollution (like syphilis), created a precedent for understanding AIDS through and beyond stigma (104–5). Emily Martin, in her 1994 monograph, *Flexible Bodies: Tracking Immunity in American Culture from the Days of Polio to the Age of AIDS*, makes important connections between shifting understandings of the immune system as a fortress in the mid-twentieth century to the immune system as a flexible and adaptable complex of systems in light of immunology research and the HIV crisis and our understandings of economic systems; for Martin, economic ideas transfer to biological systems. Legal scholars, such as Ruth Colker, have written about the contested relationship between disability activists and HIV activists during the drafting of the Americans with Disability Act, with disability activists distancing themselves from those living with HIV (Colker 22–65 2005); it was not until *Bragdon v. Abbott* in 1998 (eighteen years after the crisis in the US began) that people with asymptomatic HIV became covered under the Americans with Disability Act (US Supreme Court).

8. Stigma is perhaps most famously theorized by Irving Goffman as a trait, behavior, or reputation—one to be seen as abnormal—that causes one to be rejected by a social group (131–40).

9. I am also deeply indebted to a generation of disability studies scholars who took up Goffman; the 2014 *Disability Studies Quarterly* forum "Reflections on the Fiftieth Anniversary of Erving Goffman's *Stigma*" is particularly helpful for understanding how Goffman's work itself has circulated and been critiqued. Please see *Disability Studies Quarterly* vol. 34, no. 1, 2014, edited by Rosemarie Garland-Thomson and Jeffrey Brune.

ity life writing: how a book is marketed, in addition to how an author writes about her own relationship to writing and income, affects readers' interpretations of the value of the narrative. As we will understand in the chapters that follow, mediated author–reader relationships produce an economy of relation that reinforces stigma for the HIV subject and ultimately affects how a person living with HIV is afforded medical care. However, not all author–reader relationships produce the same outcome; women living with HIV reading the experience of authors living with HIV provides space for alternative interpretations that can raise the political consciousness of readers, leading to readers developing more agency in advocating for appropriate medical care. The political economy of stigma operates anticipating one reader response that can shore up medical and social institutions. Those marginalized by intersectional systems of oppression, however, can provide us strategies for offering and receiving narratives in resistance to the political economy of stigma.

Narrative and Medicine

There is a rise in interest in disability life writing, both in the publication industry and in the medical industry.[10] In the 1980s and 1990s, the personal and political experience of HIV/AIDS sparked a number of narratives that challenged cultural scripts (Couser 2006, 399). Disability theorist G. Thomas Couser argues that the memoir boom, theorized by Smith and Watson as a publication and reading trend in the last decades of the twentieth century, is a disability life-writing boom, what Couser himself terms *autosomatography* (2009, 2, 164).[11] While Couser's seminal work in disability life narra-

---

10. While a comprehensive history of disability life writing has yet to be written, disability theorist Thomas Couser marks the era right after World War II as the beginning of the genre, stemming from both disabled veterans and the polio epidemic (2006, 399). We could also trouble this limited understanding of life writing if we were to think about how published narrative accompanied freak-show exhibitions (see Robert Bogdan, "The Social Construction of Freaks," *Freakery: Cultural Spectacles of the Extraordinary Body* [New York UP, 1996], pp. 23–38; and Rosemarie Garland-Thomson, "Introduction: From Wonder to Error—A Genealogy of Freak Discourse in Modernity," in the same volume) or if we were to look at mendicant literature (see Susan Schweik, *The Ugly Laws: Disability in Public* [New York UP, 2009]), both dating back to the mid-1800s. This would also expand racial and class representation of disability literature.

11. For Couser, what makes this new upsurge unique is the memoir's "disability consciousness"; in other words, the rhetorical move itself of focusing on the disability versus the impairment (2009, 165). Despite these rhetorical developments in the new disability memoir, Couser laments that an intersectional analysis of disability is unusual (176) and that the disability memoir as a whole still represents a primarily White, middle-class authorship (190). Theorizing disability life writing from HIV memoir provides a more nuanced and intersectional interpretation of disability and life writing as a whole.

tive provides an important foundation for this project, this project diverges from Couser's by using a feminist disability studies analysis. I propose that we understand disability life writing as both a material product from which medical and publication industries benefit and an ideological product central to neoliberal governance. This neoliberal governance works through the political economy of stigma, which reifies systems of oppression and privilege by appropriating and interpreting narratives by and about disabled people.

Disability studies scholars such as Chris Bell and Achim Nowak have productively written about processes of HIV disclosure—to sexual partners, workplaces, and medical communities (Bell; Nowak). In questioning the apparatuses of disclosure, both scholars have highlighted systems and structures that contribute to the biopolitical regulation of HIV; this project extends those analyses by working through *how* disclosure circulates as a compulsory mechanism of the political economy of stigma. In my research with women living with HIV, I interrogate disclosure at a few levels: the first is the process of my research participants' disclosures to me, which they all weave into a story of paid work and career; second, I analyze my participants' disclosures in the workplace and their personal lives—how and when they deem disclosure necessary; finally, I analyze how disclosure itself functions as a tool for medical subservience and, at times, medical abuse.

This project resists the idea that personal narrative about illness or disability is supplemental. Lisa Diedrich asks, "How do illness narratives (by patients but also by doctors) supplement the stories of disease, diagnosis, and cure articulated within the institutional and epistemological frameworks of medicine? At the same time, how do illness narratives inevitably fail to articulate the whole story of illness?" (2007, 83). Diedrich begins with an understanding of personal narrative as contingent on the hegemonic medical diagnosis—indeed, can the medical be the supplemental to the personal? I suggest a reversal—that personal narrative can stand independent of the medical. In doing so, I question this idea of a narrative failure. Is a narrative a failure because it does not meet medical expectations, as Diedrich suggests? Or because it does not encapsulate all of one's experience?[12] My research moves beyond this configuration of failure/success in order to take seriously how medicine itself produces several kinds of reading strategies.

This project also works from the assumption that illness and disability narratives are not a de facto interruption of the power of medicine. Disability studies and medical humanities scholars such as Rosemarie Garland-

---

12. Thanks to an anonymous peer reviewer for providing another way to understand this excerpt. Irony of context accepted.

Thomson, Arthur Frank, and Lisa Diedrich have argued that "illness narratives can produce and reflect 'a *radical democratization of medicine*'" (Diedrich 3); the problem with this articulation is that it assumes that what one writes will be received with the same intention. If we understand experience itself as reflective of a negotiation of power, and one's ability to receive another's experience as reflective of similar power negotiations, then we can begin to unpack how one negotiates narrative depending on their own reading of these relations. The political economy of stigma is a social regulation of belonging and participation seen through the circulation and reception of life narratives within a neoliberal political context; if neoliberalism is a system of political organization that values individualism, profit, and globalization, then the circulation of life narratives becomes a way to bolster these systems through both the material and the ideological production of stigma.

Similar to Frank and Diedrich, Rebecca Garden has argued that "much of the medical humanities' focus has been trained on the experience of the individual—in pointed opposition to biomedicine's diseases, disorders and populations—and this discipline has emphasized narrative as a necessary and neglected dimension of data" (2015, 77). I do not disagree with Garden on the importance of addressing narratives to personalize the experience of illness for medical professionals; however, I do want to caution us against removing the attention to "diseases, disorders and populations" in our consideration of these texts. We need to continue to consider "diseases, disorders and populations" in order to understand HIV memoir, for instance, but we can read these memoirs not as indicative of individual failure or triumph but as a way to understand institutional oppression and the circulation of stigma. The political economy of stigma asks us to hold personal narrative in relation to diseases, disorders, and populations because this triad provides a ground on which we interpret and find narratives valuable within a neoliberal economy. This triad is how narratives get made accessible in the first place—providing a generic frame within which they circulate. A feminist disability studies approach to personal narrative must be concerned with processes and effects of diagnosis. Eli Clare reminds us: "Diagnosis wields immense power. It can provide us access to vital medical technology or shame us, reveal a path toward less pain or get us locked up" (41). Diagnosis (and cures) are tools of power that organize our realities (41). We must read narratives in relation to diagnosis, sometimes skeptical, sometimes curious, sometimes relieved.

Because personal narratives about illness and disability cannot be read without a relationship to diagnosis, we must understand these texts as theoretical texts for the practice of medicine. Garden argues that "making these autobiographical texts central to theory and pedagogy is a way of advocating on behalf of the authors and these categories of people they represent, those who have less power and privilege in the clinical setting and in society because they are ill and disabled and may have other marginalized identities or social conditions" (2015, 77). I take Garden's premise a step further by centering the textual and paratextual contexts of these autobiographical texts in terms of the political economy of stigma, so that the analysis of power between the author and reader is not only supplemental to the reading of the text and the creation of theory; the analysis of power *is* the theory. Thus, the political economy of stigma asks us not to see the inclusion of personal narrative in medical training or practice as advocating for marginalized people; it asks us to unpack how the mechanisms of marginality work in the first place. These texts are not ways to advocate *for* marginalized people; when we unveil the mechanisms of marginalization, we can better understand how it is that oppressed people are advocating for themselves through creating and sharing critical social theory. The political economy of stigma deepens Garden's call to situate our "own knowledge and agency, as well as the conditions of representation at work in any given narrative," including understanding the "pressures of the book market" (80). The political economy of stigma provides us the theoretical apparatus to unpack how personal agency and knowledge are conditioned and circulated within a neoliberal economy, including the pressures of the book market and the influences of the medical industrial complex.

Additionally, my project understands illness itself as an event. Diedrich proposes that illness narratives can be understood as "symptomatic texts of our time" both because they describe symptoms and, more importantly, because they "describe illness as an event that goes beyond any particular individual's experience and account of it" (2007, vii). Like Diedrich's, my project takes seriously the knowledges produced within HIV memoir as expert knowledges; unlike Diedrich, I am interested not in psychoanalytic approaches to these texts but in how these texts, both in their writing and in their circulation, produce a conceptualization of citizenship for those with chronic illness. My research within contemporary HIV narratives demonstrates how some categories of identification become available for some women living with HIV and remain unavailable to others; how some readers are socially situated to identify with texts and others to identify against. While Diedrich herself distinguishes between "good memoir and bad memoir (and everything in between)" (xv), I resist any kind of binary but instead ask how some memoir is politically produced to resonate with dominant White middle-class values and others are not. A distinction between "good" and "bad" reinforces the hegemonic knowledge-making that this project seeks to unravel. Diedrich writes, "Illness provides a phenomenological reduction of sorts that allows one to look anew upon that which one has formerly taken for granted, in terms of one's relationship to the world, to others, and to the self" (xviiii). This articulation risks a romanticization of illness itself, one that relies on a firm "before," which, as Angela Carter astutely reminds us in her work on trauma, is much more difficult for multiply marginalized people. If illness, like trauma, is just one of many marginalizing events, as many of the women I worked with articulated for themselves, then this idea of "before" becomes a murky point in time. So, what, indeed, happens on a subjective and intersubjective level, as Diedrich proposes, if the self is politically mobile in the first place? This book explores just that, arguing that the self is mobilized through a political economy of stigma that reinforces systems of oppression and privilege, particularly in relation to the medical industrial complex, preventing possibilities for transforming care for those most stigmatized.

Narrative Ethics

This project provides three critiques: of illness narratives (specifically HIV narratives); of reading practices themselves (informed by those who provide medical treatments and social services for those living with HIV); and of educational and professional practices (specifically narrative medicine) within the medical humanities that use illness narratives to improve medical practice.

From the beginning, I have paid careful attention to the ethics of my project: If I was going to be engaging narrative as a scholar, how could I ensure that I would not recreate the very practices I critique? That I, myself, would not participate in the production and circulation of stigma for those living with HIV or for those who provide medical care? What if, in calling attention to the mechanisms of stigma that those living with HIV experience, I move the stigma from HIV patient to HIV care provider? Can I myself write anything as a scholar within the academe without acquiring a smug, all-knowing, self-righteous persona?

Perhaps ironically, in 2004 disability life-writing theorist G. Thomas Couser turned to biomedicine's ethics—respect for autonomy, nonmaleficence, beneficence, and justice—to propose an ethics to life writing more broadly (he was not simply referring to life writing about illness and disability) (14–33). Key for Couser is the relationship between the subject and the reader, as well as an acknowledgment that the more vulnerable the subject of life writing, the higher the ethical stakes (19). Couser proposes the need for transparency between writer and subject as well as between writer and reader.

Stigma intentionally obscures this transparent relationship; using the theoretical apparatus of the political economy of stigma can help unveil these relationships between author and reader. Throughout my writing in this monograph, I remain clear with the readers about the research process, just as, throughout my research process, I remained clear with my research participants about my writing project. In these pages, I tell the story of the research.

I have also asked myself about the suitability and accessibility of writing for academia: would my research participants ever be able to access this writing? This speaks to a central point of tension in doing feminist disability studies work itself. While this monograph may not be accessible to all participants, the theories my participants helped me construct have led to ongoing projects beyond this particular book: for example, the group of women living with HIV continued to meet and form programming after the formal research ended; in coalition with the AIDS service worker group, I have begun collecting and archiving oral histories in a publicly accessible digital archive. In many ways, these projects are, too, part of this story even though they fall outside these pages.

In remaining transparent with readers, telling the story of this research begins with the central belief I had about *why* HIV, *why* women, *why* now. I believed in the beginning that writing about the experience of HIV thirty years after the crisis in the US began would shed light on mechanisms of medicine that need improvement as well as mechanisms of medicine and care that work well.

I also believed that humanities theories, particularly those invested in a feminist and social justice politic, could help us all make sense of systems of oppression within medical care. I still believe this to be true, even as my understandings of these mechanisms and theories have evolved. My project has been affected by the critical interventions of health humanities scholar Delese Wear, who in 1992 is one of the first scholars in medicine to ask us to think critically about the medical humanities themselves, both in what we do as scholars and in how we teach as pedagogues. Wear asks us, in bringing the humanities into medical classrooms and medical practice, to not "mimic what we perceive to be the methods or postures of science" and to instead embrace a postmodern approach that recognizes "our knowing as inevitably and always partial, positioned, culture-bound and perspectival" (201). Wear asks us not to look for a core truth in our practices with patient-clients and students and to resist positioning ourselves as "Grand Theorists," purveyors of privileged knowledge. She asks us, as have feminist theorists before her (notably, she references bell hooks, Audre Lorde, and Patti Lather), to make explicit our political commitments (205–9). Thus, in my relationship with research participants and within my writing itself, I strive for transparency—to tell my participants what my project is about and why I am seeking their help, to share with my readers significant portions of original transcriptions to provide room for them to interpret for themselves, even as I provide my own theoretical interpretations.

Tale of Two Reading Groups

With five HIV memoirs as a scaffold, this book draws on original research in two different reading groups: one group with women living with HIV during the period 2012–13; a second group with AIDS service workers in 2015. Both groups are located in two different midsize rust-belt cities not often considered to be centers of HIV activism. I selected a population of women living with HIV because these women move in and out of experiencing debilitating bodily conditions, changing their relationship to disability daily. Because little has been written about HIV memoir in academic and popular settings, reading about HIV gives more room for creative and alternative interpretations than reading about other kinds of stigmatized illness. I also wanted to work with AIDS service workers to find whether their experience of reading HIV memoirs contrasted the experience of women living with HIV; as a group of medical practitioners, AIDS service workers tend to have a more political orientation than other practitioners, many having begun their work because of HIV stigma and injustice in the 1980s and early 1990s. Having groups in two separate cities was important because participants in each group would not directly know participants in the other and feel unable to speak candidly. Both groups read a selection of HIV memoirs (choosing from the five that serve as the project scaffolding) and other popular disability memoirs over the course of several months.[13] By working with my research participants in this way, we were able to form a longer-term relationship built on trust; the memoirs also worked as a conduit for inspiring conversation topics and personal disclosures that I believe would not have been revealed in shorter, more direct interviews or focus groups. Through my research I found that central to both groups' understandings of stigma and illness are conceptualizations of labor and medical citizenship.

This project is not the first to think critically about spectatorship, reader reception, and oppression. Perhaps most notably for readers of this monograph, bell hooks writes about oppositional spectatorship, expanding the work

---

13. See Appendix A for reading group lists.

of Stuart Hall and Franz Fanon, writing, "Subordinates in relations of power learn experientially that there is a critical gaze, one that 'looks' to document, one that is oppositional. In resistance struggle, the power of the dominated to assert agency by claiming and cultivating 'awareness' politicizes looking relations—one learns to look a certain way in order to resist" (95). In other words, writing from her own experience as a Black woman viewing/receiving White media, hooks tells us that how we receive media productions depends on where we are sitting in relation to oppression and privilege—and if we are experiencing oppression, our reception is one attuned to operations of power. Our reception is oppositional. Our reception is perhaps unintended or unpredictable. Lauren Berlant writes, in her oft-cited article "The Female Complaint" (and expands this in her book by the same title), that even if we are all members of one oppressed group—in her examples, women—we must not be expected to share a single reception; to borrow bell hooks's phrase, there is no single oppositional gaze. In her critique, Berlant asks us to understand the public sphere as simply the place where the dominant group(s) makes and enforces meaning (240). Others make meaning in the shadows of these spheres, and their work, in Berlant's context specifically female sentimental culture of soap operas and romance novels, serves as a "safety valve" for "surplus female rage and desire" (245). The work by oppressed groups is not taken seriously by dominant culture, but Berlant is one of the many feminist scholars to ask us to understand the political importance of these safety valves, slowly turning them to release multiple deluges against patriarchal dominance. Julie Elman expands work on spectatorship and citizenship by writing about popular culture and teenagers in the twentieth century, proposing that popular teen dramas are doing more than simply promoting sentimental, vacuous entertainment; they are creating understandings of teenagers themselves as disabled adults and "edutainment" as necessary rehabilitation, all while promoting neoliberal, heterosexual able-bodied citizenship (1–27). What is produced by dominant culture for popular entertainment must be understood both as a safety valve to contain oppositional spectatorship and as a producer of that spectatorship. Unintended receptions are part and parcel of how the political economy of stigma works, creating meaning through one's relationship to oppression and privilege.

While hooks, Elman, and Berlant have been influential for this monograph, the methodology for this research has two strong influences. The first is Janice Radway's groundbreaking *Reading the Romance: Women, Patriarchy, and Popular Literature*. Like Radway, I am interested in the reception of popular narratives; the memoirs that we read would not be considered "elite literature" (3), and, like the romance industry in the 1980s that Radway analyzes, these memoirs are marketed through a political economy that takes to its advantage changing publication techniques (19–45).[14] Like Radway, I place the production of memoir in the context of its political economy; books do not exist in a vacuum but are produced with audiences and commerce in mind. Yet, my research differs from Radway's in two significant ways: first, the memoirs I analyze alongside my reading group participants are not all geared toward a popular, middle-class audience; second, the research groups I work with are not part of a pre-existing reading group but instead were brought together for the purpose of this research. Thus, not only does this change the way my research participants relate to one another, but most of my research participants were not initially interested in the reading material analyzed here. Some were not frequent readers at all; others read the occasional novel (Harry Potter) or other *New York Times* bestsellers. As part of my analysis in the following chapters, I discuss all of my research participants' relationships to reading prior to the research.

I have also been influenced by Megan Sweeney's research on incarcerated women's reading practices, *Reading Is My Window: Books and the Art of Reading in Women's Prisons*. Like Radway, Sweeney is interested in women's reception; unlike Radway, Sweeney does not engage women through a particular genre. Sweeney explores how women use what is available in their prison libraries to make meaning in their own lives (1–15, 173–212). Through Sweeney's careful discussion of her research participants' negotiation of (Christian) self-help books, we learn the difference between writer and publisher intent and reader reception. Sweeney writes: "Some women prisoners use reading as a means to develop their sense of agency and responsibility, change their way of thinking, reoccupy the present, and craft their life stories as more open-ended tales of becoming, opening themselves to future possibilities even when those possibilities remain circumscribed by prison bars" (212). In many ways, the women with whom Sweeney worked resisted the intent of Christian publishers while continuing to find the act of reading meaningful. Sweeney's analysis reinforces my understanding that books are always dialogic; to that end, I understood, as I was reading disability and HIV memoir, that audiences would create meanings from and through their own experiences and that perhaps the most marginalized of audiences might have the most transformative interpretations.

---

14. Radway references the kinds of glue that make mass-market paperbacks economical to produce, as well as the advent of the big-box bookstore, as changing the landscape of reading culture; we might be able to make similar arguments about memoir and the proliferation of self-publishing and e-book publishing today.

Perhaps to the readers of this scholarly monograph, these divergent recep-tions of memoir will not be surprising. And yet, I hesitate to think that there is one reaction of readers at all—to this project or any other. There must always be multiple receptions to any project, and the political economy of stigma is one way we might understand this differentialness. We might say that the political economy of stigma is a theory about citizenship and reading, creating feelings of belonging along and through vectors of oppression and privilege.

Praxis and Interpretation

My research here is first and foremost a close reading of narrative—both pub-lished written narrative and oral narrative collected here for the first time. This project follows contemporary theories in feminist autobiographical studies in recognizing that autobiography itself is an open-ended history of embodi-ment. As Susannah Mintz writes, "Disability is an inconstant experience, its significance to the story of self, requiring multiple retellings, repeated narra-tive shaping" (4). While I believe the narratives I analyze here share themes of disabled embodiment, intersectional oppression, and an ongoing negotia-tion of medical power relations with other disability narratives, particularly those narratives that address chronic illness, there is also a way in which this research highlights the particular and not the universal.

This research is not meant to speak for all people living with HIV or for all medical practitioners working with people living with HIV; if one were to replicate this research, they might find similar themes and accounts but also important differences. The project of theorizing through and alongside nar-rative is intended to bring to the fore marginalized experiences while main-taining keen attention to the power relations that shape those experiences. Feminist theorist Sara Ahmed asks us to question how some texts become considered theory and others not, and how systems of power play into those demarcations (8–10). Ahmed writes that "we use the particulars to challenge the universal" (10), and, indeed, this project is doing just that: the broadest particular is the experience of HIV in the US as understood through pub-lished life writing and my own ethnographic work with reading HIV and dis-ability memoir with women living with HIV. These forms of life story, in the repeatings and retellings and contradictions, are embodied theory about iden-tity, self, illness, and citizenship; I read them as such.

This project is rooted in practices of close reading with attention to inter-sectional power dynamics and social justice. I begin by conducting a close reading of published memoirs written by women living with HIV in the US.

I then turn to the transcripts of two different groups of people with whom I engaged about these memoirs—one a group of women living with HIV, the other a co-ed group of HIV service workers. Finally, I analyze the documents and discourses of narrative medicine at Columbia University, a fast-growing training mechanism for medical practitioners. My analysis consists of closely reading core texts of narrative medicine, analyzing my own experience in a weekend narrative medicine workshop, and tracing the adoption of narrative medicine as both a brand and a practice in other publication venues. Because of the operation of the political economy of stigma, narrative medicine is not able to accomplish what it set out to do—to address the social justice concerns in the practice of medicine; moreover, it may actually be doing harm.

Analyzing published HIV narratives written by women in the US, their reception by women living with HIV and AIDS practitioners, and the increasing development of medical humanities programs such as narrative medicine that have an interest in collecting life narratives in order to address structural problems within medical practice itself, all serve to illustrate precisely how the political economy of stigma works as a strategy of neoliberal governmentality. My ethnographic analysis reveals a disturbing trend in the medical field's uptake of disability life narratives (a broad term encompassing published and unpublished narrative, written, digital, and spoken) that medical practitioners risk reinforcing harmful stigmas that draw on underlying notions of deserving and undeserving citizens when they circulate patient narratives. While there is potential to transform the health humanities through narrative, taking lessons from narrative medicine scholars like Sayantani DasGupta (whom I address in my conclusion), I ultimately argue that while the political economy of stigma remains in operation, the appropriation of narrative by medical practitioners will only ever be one more location within which the political economy of stigma is operationalized.

In this project I explore the difference between medical practitioner attention to narrative and medical practitioner appropriation of patient narrative, understanding that not all attention to narrative within medicine is misguided or nefarious. Within the political economy of stigma, medical appropriation of personal narrative eliminates the transformative potential of personal narrative through disenfranchising those "patients" with whom they collaborate.

While I am critical of narrative appropriation within medical practice, I am also deeply committed to understanding the transformative potential that narrative can provide. Thus, my investigations in this project are shaped by ethical considerations of "vulnerable subjects" (Couser 2004, xii).[15] I spent

---

15. Couser explores the relationship of medicine to narrative in a book-length treatment, *Vulnerable Subjects: Ethics and Life Writing*, of which I say more in chapter 2. For now, I highlight how Couser defines vulnerable subjects, "persons who are liable to exposure by someone

hours discussing feminist ethics for this project with faculty advisors, peer mentors, ethics board personnel, and community members in HIV service work. As a White queer invisibly disabled women not living with HIV, I thought carefully about how to work with people living with HIV, how and when to begin the project, what kinds of compensation would be ethical for participants, and what explanations I could provide about the project's goals. My conversations clarified my own expectations, which were open-ended: I needed the perspectives of those affected by HIV (both those living with and care providers) to unpack and analyze with me the HIV memoirs I was reading. The books themselves provided a buffer for our conversation—a conduit through which participants could, if they chose, share their personal experience. The vulnerability and needs of my research participants did not just inform my approach to the research; my understanding of their vulnerability *was* my approach to the research. They, in turn, responded to my transparency as we analyzed texts together, told our own life stories, and responded to one another's summaries and contradictions. Feminist disability research requires an engagement with vulnerable subjects, and by beginning with an understanding of that vulnerability and being transparent with all research participants about the process of research and writing, I created an ethical contract with my participants that was reinforced by formal ethical review boards.

Recruiting for this project was a tricky experience; for my first research group, with women living with HIV, I encountered several barriers, explained briefly below, and ultimately worked with three women in the reading group over six months. In recruiting my second group with AIDS service workers, I collaborated with established networks of care providers; I ultimately facilitated a group with six participants. Neither group is meant to be a positivist account of what all women living with HIV experience or what all AIDS service workers experience; instead, as a feminist disability methodologist, I sought, first, to theorize alongside those with embodied experiences and, second, to collect life narratives not just from those with the privilege of access to publication. Thus, I include large excerpts throughout the book of my participants' own words, choosing to allow these excerpts to stand on their own for reader interpretation; I follow these excerpts with theoretical models that are helpful for interpreting these narratives but do not weave the theory heavily into my participants' narratives. This is my attempt to honor my participants' contributions while also guiding readers through my own interpretations of their narratives. I trust that readers here will bring their own models of interpretation.

---

with whom they are involved in an intimate or trust-based relationship but are unable to represent themselves in writing or to offer meaningful consent to their representation by someone else" (xii).

I first used the networks I knew through my own long-term weekly volunteer work to recruit women for a reading group, working with two significant ASOs, one freestanding and one connected to a regional children's hospital. I also presented my research program on two different occasions to a coalition of state ASOs at their monthly meeting. I received the most support for the project, and all of my participants, through the networks at the freestanding ASO, probably because the staff knew me as a long-term volunteer. I heard quite a bit of resistance to my project at the regional children's hospital ASO; as one long-term, White social work employee responded, "Our women are not readers. I think this is going to be over their heads. They are Hispanic."[16] While I certainly cannot assume that everyone in the room believed what this social worker voiced, I can tell you that no one spoke up against this assumption about literacy or interest but merely nodded their heads in agreement. Although I made many follow-up phone calls and emails and emphasized the accommodations I could provide (audio books, for instance), the program at the children's hospital never responded to my recruitment efforts.

As I was recruiting, I wrote grants to fund the program (funds that provided books and food) and did more recruiting in networks that I was much less familiar with (for instance, I sent 150 mailers to Black churches, advertising the program). I then conducted initial interviews, which asked about everything from reading practices (to assess literacy levels of participants— if they could read a copy of the local paper, they could read the memoirs selected for the group) to history with HIV.[17] In this initial interview, I was clear with each participant that I was not a woman living with HIV myself but that I had been affected by HIV in my personal life. I also made it clear that I identified as having another disability and welcomed questions.[18]

---

16. I formally presented at the regional children's hospital meeting for HIV care providers on September 12, 2012. There were thirteen social workers and health-care workers present.

17. The women living with HIV reading group was approved by the IRB of the institution with which I was associated at the time of the research; the AIDS service worker reading group, as well as my participant observation of Columbia University's Narrative Medicine workshop, was given exemption from the IRB of the institution with which I was associated at the time of research.

18. I in no way interacted with participants outside my reading groups, I had no preexisting relationships with participants when the groups began, and I have not continued relationships outside of my role as a researcher with any group participants. While my facilitation style was friendly, there was never any confusion about my being a researcher. This was made clear with the reading of oral consent prior to every meeting, by the visible presence of a tape recorder throughout sessions, and by my professional reminder phone calls prior to each meeting. I also only ever emailed participants from my professional university email address. All meetings also took place within professional AIDS service worker conference rooms; a few interviews with AIDS service workers whom I screened for participation took place outside of nine-to-five office hours at a local public coffee shop.

I worked through similar networks in my second city when I began recruiting for AIDS service workers. I began by contacting the regional affiliate of the ASO that I had worked with previously, the local Ryan White program, and the local public health office. I was invited to recruit at staff meetings at two ASOs and recruited six participants. In Part II and Part III, I most directly address the life experiences of those in both reading groups, theorizing power dynamics in local communities that make some more available to participate in research than others.

All participants knew that I was writing a book about these reading groups and frequently asked me when I would have the material ready for the book as the reading groups progressed. I mentioned that the writing and publishing process would take years following the conclusion of our time together; all participants understood that they would not read a final product. I was consistently honored by disclosures of participants but never directly asked them to disclose personal details. My discussion of the one-on-one interview responses to questions about why one would write a memoir, and what effect the reading group had on individual lives, is pertinent to understanding why participants were drawn to the project in the first place. Participating in the project helped us all think about the vulnerabilities of publishing personal narrative, including as part of an academic study.

For the women living with HIV in my first group, while we were reading, they disidentified with disability while simultaneously claiming HIV as central to their identity; at the same time, their negotiations of neglectful and abusive medical systems served as a source of solidarity and identification with disability activists. As queer theorist José Muñoz has written, disidentification is a strategy of minoritarian subjects (for Muñoz, queer people of color, but, more broadly, any subject occupying multiply marginalized positionalities) to interpret dominant representations in such a way that one neither fully conforms to nor fully resists those representations (4, 12–25). Feminist disability theorist Sami Schalk has extended Muñoz to crip theory, writing:

> Taking up this adapted understanding of disidentification, I find myself, a minoritarian subject, disidentifying with disability studies, a minoritarian field of research, because although the field's resistance to the pathologization of non-normative bodies appeals to me as a nondisabled, fat, black, queer woman, the shortage of substantive race analysis within the field and the relatively minor attention given to issues of class and sexuality trouble me deeply and disallow me any direct Good Subject identification.

For Schalk, disidentification opens up a place for identifying with crip, "an almost-not-quite-yet-identification" and a means for building coalitional political praxis. I believe that the women living with HIV with whom I worked similarly claim a disidentification with disability; for them, this is a reading strategy, a resource access strategy, and, ultimately, a survival strategy.

While the women in this reading group did not identify as "having" a disability when our group began, they did access disability-related resources as a result of their HIV diagnosis. They also all experienced workplace and medical discrimination. Through their labor of reading and writing about medical negotiations by both women living with HIV and women living with other disability, the women in my first reading group engaged in a differential citizenship that reimagines the self through and beyond medical labor and provides a new epistemology for understanding disability identification. I am using *differential* here in the tradition of critical cultural theorist Chela Sandoval to mean critical and mobile; Sandoval uses this term to apply to a consciousness of oppressed people who navigate between and among various forms of oppression and enact this consciousness in relation to their understandings of power. In adapting Sandoval's term to apply to reader reception, I am reinforcing the importance of readers' negotiations of power as an act of reading.

For the participants in my second reading group, who were all AIDS service workers and understood themselves as activists prior to their engagement in AIDS service work, their labor as AIDS service workers became a primary identification. Through their labor, they, too, understood the stickiness of stigma; they were often assumed to be living with the virus themselves because of their deep association with their work. For those who also identified as gay men, their experience was especially sticky.[19] Unlike the women in my first reading group who claimed solidarity with disability activists, AIDS service workers in my second reading group reinforced neoliberal models of self and other, doctor / social worker and patient, in their reimagining of themselves through medical labor. These distinct understandings of engaged citizenship through medical labor led to divergent receptions of the same HIV memoirs, leading to the central argument of this project: that the act of reading and writing illness relies on a negotiation of labor and medical citizenship that can be best understood by analyzing the formal and informal negotiations of narrative and citizenship within the political economy of stigma.

---

19. This claim of HIV identity is perhaps similar to Robert McRuer's disclosures of wearing an HIV-positive T-shirt while having a seronegative status (57), which led to some controversy about crip identification; this practice of McRuer's was later theorized by Victoria Kannen as indicative of a "post-identarian space" (159).

Chapter Summaries

In part I, "The Neoliberalizing of Narrative," my chapters are linked together with this idea that memoir circulates as a commodity and has explicit material effects. In these first two chapters, I present the problem of why the current circulation of illness and disability memoir does not address issues of social justice. I begin in chapter 1, "The Political Economy of Stigma and the Production of Memoir," by addressing the political economy of HIV memoir (the memoir industry), a genre of life writing that reinforces ideas of deserving and undeserving citizens within neoliberalism. Once I establish disability life writing as a form of governmentality, I provide a genealogy of HIV life writing by women in the US, a genealogy that begins more than fifteen years into the HIV epidemic there. I argue that women's voices emerge in this epidemic in relation to welfare reform and to what Ange-Marie Hancock calls the politics of disgust; in order to understand how these narratives are operating in relation to the politics of disgust, I analyze what kinds of presses produce and circulate HIV memoir written by women. Finally, in this chapter, I ask my reading groups to reflect on why they think HIV memoir is written and produced, analyzing how the neoliberal market and individual publishers can anticipate reader interpretation but not limit it. The political economy of stigma allows us to understand the sophisticated relationships between authors and readers that develop in relation to medicine, markets, and public policy.

In chapter 2, "Writing Labor, Writing Privilege in HIV Memoir," I conduct a close reading of themes of labor in three memoirs read by my reading groups as well as my participants' reactions to them. In addition to discussing Hoffman and Wyatt-Morley, I analyze a memoir written by Paula Peterson; this memoir is the winner of a literary prize and is marketed to a more literary audience through muted colors on the cover art and an academic press. All three women are writing about their experience with HIV during the same period, and yet their understanding of illness is racialized: Peterson writes reinforcing stereotypes of the "welfare queen" in order to claim a kind of remarkability as a White mother with HIV and to gain reader sympathy. This difference in reception to these three memoirs, a pattern between my two reading groups, highlights the importance of how a memoir is marketed in addition to how the memoirists understand themselves as part of an HIV political economy.[20]

---

20. When thinking about political economy in relation to disability and/or illness, I am indebted to the work of scholar-activist Marta Russell for her analysis of how disabled bodies contribute to the political economics of neoliberalism in the period directly following the pass-

In part II, "The Privilege of Privacy," I explore how the political economy of stigma problematizes the use of narrative within medicine. I draw on Black feminist scholars and their articulations of privacy to question the utility of narrative within medicine. As Black feminist scholar Karla Holloway tells us, privacy is a privilege that has not been afforded to women or to people of color; we see this negation of privacy in the interactions of medical practitioners that demand unnecessary details from women living with HIV and reinforce historical patterns of oppression through HIV stigma. In chapter 3, "Diagnostic Reading and the Limits of Disability Memoir," I capture the reading practices and conversations with one group of AIDS service workers, analyzing a pattern of reception that I call *diagnostic reading*. Diagnostic reading is a practice of reading where readers consciously or unconsciously read for problem-solving a memoirist's disclosures as symptoms of an overarching medical diagnosis. In the process, they individualize sociopolitical and structural oppression, and limit the transformative potential of disclosure for social and medical justice. This is how the political economy of stigma operates. We might understand diagnostic reading and the political economy of stigma as a component crucial to feminist disability theorist Julie Elman's model of rehabilitative citizenship, where "the emphasis on individual health empowerment" transforms the call for redistribution of resources to those least empowered into "corporate profits—soothing and profiting from an anxiety felt by many in an age of increasingly precarious relationships to economic security and access to health insurance and care" (174). One need not be a trained medical practitioner to produce a pattern of diagnostic reading themselves; similarly, not all medical practitioners are diagnostic readers.

In chapter 4, "Privacy, Bioethics, and Narrative Medicine," I address the brand of narrative medicine as one site where narrative is used as part of a pedagogical practice to teach empathy and social justice issues within medicine. I argue, however, that because of the political economy of stigma, narrative medicine risks reifying stigma for those with chronic disabling conditions. This chapter includes my personal experience, my own narrative of narrative medicine conferences, to form a metacritique of the practice using their own tools of close reading and writing.

In part III, "Beyond the Parallel Chart," I propose ways to crip memoir in medical practices, moving beyond narrative medicine's parallel chart to contextualize experiences of illness and diagnosis within larger systems of structural oppression. In chapter 5, "Work, Disclosure, and the HIV Origin Story,"

---

ing of the ADA; I am also indebted to the earlier work of Deborah Stone, who theorizes how the government and medicine work together to produce the administrative category of disability.

I return to the analysis of women living with HIV, my first reading group, all of whom disclosed their own HIV origin stories in the context of paid work and discrimination. I capture these origin stories here as a starting place for transforming and cripping the use of personal narrative—the chapter questions how and why my research participants frame their HIV diagnosis within an analysis of work and related structural oppressions.

In chapter 6, "Power, Resistance, and Differential Reading Practices," my reading group of AIDS service workers provides me a key reading practice, one that I call *differential reading,* extending Chela Sandoval's conceptualization of differential consciousness in *Methodology of the Oppressed.* Differential reading is a practice I witnessed among women living with HIV that was dialogic; differential reading provides us a framework for reading narratives within medicine not with a positivist intent on diagnosis but with a transformational and contingent analysis of power. One way that power operates in the lives of women with HIV is through administrative violence, a concept I borrow from critical trans scholar Dean Spade to emphasize the regulatory and mundane forms of exploitation.

In my conclusion, I analyze one final memoir, written by a young woman born with HIV, and how she creates a legible identification in a time of increasing austerity and major funding cuts through framing herself as a victim of bullying and, in these crip times, a deserving citizen-subject. In my analysis, I return to the central question of the manuscript: what would an approach to narrative and medicine look like if it used a feminist disability studies lens and method? My conclusion broadens the implications of *The Political Economy of Stigma* beyond narrative or medicine to ideologies of identity and citizenship. By making connections to what Ellen Samuels terms *biocertification,* I make a key feminist disability studies move, connecting institutional critiques to ideological systems. Here, I propose that we understand life writing within a larger practice of biocertification and what Ellen Samuels calls "fantasies of identification"; HIV life writing takes on particular significance in a time when clients accessing HIV medication through the Treatment Modernization Act (the 2006 reauthorization of the Ryan White Care Act) must submit biomedical evidence such as blood tests documenting their CD4 cell counts. Life writing is one way to both resist this classification and simplification of HIV through diagnostic testing and submit to this call for increased surveillance by medical professionals. In contrast to this surveillance, members of my first reading group provide the final narratives of analysis, providing templates for how governmental surveillance and resistance work in tension to create new models of enacting citizenship and belonging beyond the political economy of stigma.

PART I

THE NEOLIBERALIZING OF NARRATIVE

CHAPTER 1

The Political Economy of Stigma and the Production of Memoir

Neoliberalism, Narrative, and Reader Reception

Life writing, a term that encompasses a diversity of practices from tradi-
tional autobiography to more recent self-referential practices within new
media, must be understood as a tool that reinforces practices of citizenship
through the political economy of stigma.[1] As life-writing theorist Julie Rak
argues, memoir is a "citizenship technology," providing a way to express public belonging (33, 211). Extending life-writing theorists before me, I argue that
these practices of citizenship produce a political economy of stigma by mediating reader–author relationships both textually and paratextually, not just
through what one individual writes about their life experience but through
how that experience is interpreted by editors and publicists in the circulation of that narrative. All of this affects reader reception. At the same time
that memoir can be understood as a technology of citizenship, it must also be
understood as a circulating product for consumption.[2]

---

1. Marlene Kadar is the first to theorize this term precisely for its open-ended and inclusive understanding of genre; see *Essays on Life Writing: From Genre to Critical Practice* (U of
Toronto P, 1992).

2. Rak writes, "Memoir's uneasy position as a commodity and as a practice of going
public remains a way for many people to access the life and experiences of another, in order to
think through affective ties of belonging in what Lauren Berlant says we should call the affective dimensions of citizenship [. . .] Here, memoir can be viewed not as a practice of identity

One of the most popular forms of life writing is memoir about illness and disability. The mainstream public loves reading about others' experiences of disability, which is just one way that disability is commodified within, and central to, neoliberalism. Neoliberalism, which Lisa Duggan defines as "a vision of national and world order, a vision of competition, inequality, market 'discipline,' public austerity, and 'law and order,'" emerges in the 1970s through pro-business activism and broad social movement backlash (x–xi). Neoliberalism values the free market and engages in the economic project of upward redistribution and the privatization of public services over the support of a public safety net (xi–xiii). In the process of privatization, the citizen-subject of liberalism, who previously, under the liberal social contract, exchanged some freedom for the protection and services of the government, now gives up these services for the privilege of consumption; under neoliberalism, everything becomes a market product, and the citizen-subject becomes a consumer-citizen. Health care becomes one site of consumption; I argue that memoir, particularly the world of disability and illness memoir, is an essential site of consumption within neoliberal health-care models. These memoirs often focus on individual conditions, trials, and triumphs, reinforcing pity for or admiration of the individual writer at the expense of highlighting structural inequalities in health care. And they are big sellers. Julie Rak writes: "I want to change the way we have understood memoirs so that we can see them as part of a production cycle as a way to explain how the memoir boom came about, and how it continues" and emphasizes "thinking about books as commodities that are manufactured by a market for an industry" (4). As of 2002 memoir was the fourth-most-purchased book genre, with 150,000 new titles yearly (Rak 8). Another analysis suggests that sales of personal memoirs (including memoirs about childhood and memoirs about parenting) increased 400 percent during the period 2004–8 (Yagoda).

Important to understanding life writing by women with HIV is the reception of this writing; little has been written about the reception of any disability memoir, let alone HIV memoir, by people with the same or similar conditions. What do women living with HIV think about memoirs written by women living with HIV? What is the process of identification while reading these memoirs? This boom in memoirs about illness and disability demonstrates that illness and disability are actually providing theory about the self in the 1990s and 2000s that might not be developed otherwise. Disability provides an individual a heightened awareness of the body—an awareness that at once

---

in a loose sense, but as a genre that is socially produced, negotiated, negated, and embraced because technologies of identity are present within it" (213).

fractures and brings into existence a self worth writing. This self exists and provides a real lived experience for their audience to consume; the reader relies on this understanding of the real, building a relationship based on what Phillip Lejeune has called the "autobiographical pact."

When it comes to memoirs about illness and disability, health humanities scholar Rebecca Garden reminds us that the publication industry constrains how one tells their story, authors and editors "always addressing the need to tell the sort of story that will sell" (2010, 123). Garden writes: "First-person narratives in particular can seduce readers into thinking that what they read is the unmediated voice of the author, representing experience as if it were objective" (123). Additionally, Garden proposes that one might read a disability or illness narrative for "a cultural reflection of their own, sometimes isolating, experiences of disease" and would be invested in the "authenticity" of these narratives; Garden's theory importantly highlights a potential tension between the book market's motivation and the reader's motivation, whether that reader is a medical practitioner seeking an objective experience or a disabled person seeking similarities to and validation of their own experience. My research with reading groups, however, has found that this tension is productive for readers of disability and illness narratives and that contemporary readers are attuned to author and industry motivations.

To analyze any reader reception, we must first understand the role of genre and norms. As Judith Butler contends, the struggle for recognition requires a self, an other, and a readability that relies on mediated frames of reference (26–29). It is this readability that becomes most important in the production, circulation, and reception of life writing. I propose that one way to understand these mediated frames of reference is to look at the production of recognition—that is, at how a product is marketed and circulated to particular audiences. We should do this with life writing specifically.

One prominent literary studies way to understand life writing is through taxonomies; for example, theorists Smith and Watson create a taxonomy with more than sixty genres of life narrative (Rak 23). This is an incomplete and inaccurate means of theorizing life writing, for two reasons: it relies on grouping texts through diagnostic similarities such as breast cancer memoirs (mammographies),[3] which simplifies one's somatic experience as a single dominant condition (a breast cancer narrative cannot also be a depression narrative, for instance, without one condition taking precedence over another) in order to provide a satisfying narrative arc; and it relies on a static understanding of reader reception, one where the reader will prioritize one illness or

---

3. For more on published breast cancer narratives, see DeShazer; Nielsen.

condition over other themes. Many of us who teach life writing can relate to the classroom experience where we teach a memoir about, for instance, HIV; our students then surprise us by writing papers on the main character surviving domestic partner abuse, in the process never mentioning the HIV diagnosis. And yet how a memoir is categorized is what creates our expectation for the text; the HIV memoir, had it not been "about" HIV, would not have made it on to a syllabus for a class called "Disability Life Writing." Genre shapes our reader reception and interpretation, but it does not unilaterally direct it.

Genre is central to the circulation of personal narrative, shaping reader expectations within the neoliberal marketplace. Genres are exactly what allow for the circulation and recognition of a narrative; genre is about how narratives are sold to the expectations of readers (Rak 27–29). Julie Rak, the first theorist to focus on production, writes: "It is difficult to know at which point a form like memoir becomes entirely captive to market forces, or when it escapes containment and is put to previous unheard-of uses" (17–18). Like Rak, I theorize that reception is complicated. The political economy of stigma relies on genre expectations to mediate author–reader relationships. And yet, depending on the reader's relationship to medicine and illness, tropes of pity and triumph can serve to either reinforce stigma or creatively and consciously deflect it.

In my reading group research, I asked both groups—the group of women living with HIV who were clients of a local AIDS service organization and the group of ASO workers (social workers, psychiatrists, patient advocates) of a sister AIDS service organization a few hours north of the first group—for their perspective on why one might write a memoir about their experience with a disability or illness. I asked in the beginning of our meetings together, during our initial one-on-one interviews, and at the end of our time together, following several months of reading and discussion, in final one-on-one interviews. Responses indicated that the reader relates to the author of the memoir through unpacking the author's motivation, a theme that colors the ongoing discussion of the books in both reading groups.

In this chapter, I argue that the act of reading life writing itself is mediated through a political economy of stigma that can be both resisted and reinforced depending on how authors and readers situate themselves in relation to one another. Specifically, one's participation in the medical industrial complex—as a client-consumer or as a treatment provider—deeply affects how one relates to life writing about illness and disability. These relationships are mediated through a neoliberal market that anticipates a particular kind of author–reader relationality that reinforces stigma for those living with chronic illness.

To make my argument, I focus specifically on labor. I first explain disability life-writing's role within neoliberalism—what it is that life writing *does* as a product and as a form of governmentality; second, I provide a brief over-view of contemporary women's HIV memoir in the US, when and how it gets produced; third, alongside my field research participants, I analyze popu-lar expectations of HIV memoir, why individuals would write and publish a memoir that could be stigmatizing in the first place.

Life Writing and Neoliberalism

In this project about HIV life writing, I am highlighting exactly how narrative becomes included within hegemonic institutional structures such as biomedi-cine in order to reinforce a particular kind of deserving American subject. Disability studies scholars David Mitchell and Sharon Snyder argue that neo-liberal inclusionism makes newly visible identities that have been margin-alized or invisible but that, in doing so, it reifies hegemonic structures and institutions (2–3, 14): "Neoliberal marketplaces produce modern formations of disability as an increasingly malleable form of deviance tamed for the good of the nation as a potential participant in the inflows and outflows of global-ization" (17). In tandem with Mitchell and Snyder, I understand life writing as a particularly important technology of inclusionism. If we understand that neoliberal governmentality involves a "seizure of the very materiality of life at the level of the individual" (8), then we have to understand that life writing and medical storytelling are part of this governmentality—it is how we know what we are allowed to experience in relation to illness.

Tropes of inspiration and triumph have been critiqued within disability studies as providing a too individualistic understanding of disability, elimi-nating, or at least limiting, the politicization of disability. As David Mitch-ell writes, "Instead of serving as a corrective to impersonal symbolic literary representations, disability life writing tends toward the gratification of a per-sonal story bereft of community with other disabled people. Even the most renowned disability autobiographers often fall prey to an ethos of rugged indi-vidualism that can further reify the longstanding association of disability with social isolation" (312). Centering women living with HIV in an analysis of the rhetoric of disability, with an understanding of Black women in particular as made historically invisible in both the development of rhetorical theory on disability[4] and in the rising rates of HIV infection, gives us an understand-ing of how disability literature functions differently from previous scholarly interpretations.

---

4. I am grateful for the work of Stella Bolaki and Theri Pickens, who have consistently argued for returning to the work of Audre Lorde within disability studies as one way to rectify this invisibility.

Within this understanding of neoliberalism, I pay particular attention to how HIV memoirs have the potential to both produce and disrupt intersectional stigma when we analyze how memoir is circulated and marketed. How this materiality of memoir produces the political economy of stigma is precisely what I unpack below by analyzing the mediated relationships between authors and readers.

Disrupting Narrative Expectations—Women Writing HIV

No one has written about what happens to our cultural understandings of HIV from the perspective of female-bodied people as provided through published memoir. For the first fifteen years of the HIV epidemic in the US, cultural and medical understandings of HIV stemmed from male-bodied experiences that reinforce Cold War understandings of invasion. In her book-length treatment of plague texts in the era of HIV, Jacqueline Foertsch argues that many of the first HIV memoirs, written by gay men, can be understood through Cold War–era constructions of enemy, boundaries, and an ongoing apocalypse (22–24). As Foertsch writes, "The conditions prevailing during the Cold War have come to characterize the AIDS era as well, so that the body remains precariously placed and susceptible as ever to immunology's depiction of it as on the defensive yet badly defended" (23). Tracing a genealogy of plagues as considered foreign, stemming from the semen of soldiers, Sontag, like Foertsch, demonstrates how AIDS is also considered foreign (Foertsch 135–40). AIDS has been associated with primitivism and coming from the "dark continent" (140–41). Similarly, as Priscilla Wald writes of HIV in relation to other outbreak narratives, Patient 0 in the HIV narrative was understood as "alien" from the beginning (Wald 226).[5] Significant for Foertsch, Sontag, and Wald is an understanding of a barrier between "me" and "not me," between the healthy and the contagious (Foertsch 28–31).

What happens to Cold War understandings of contagion, enemies, and disease when female bodies are understood as HIV-positive? In 2010 statisticians Robert Smith and B. D. Agrawala estimate that in the US, 76.5 percent

---

5. Wald argues that "Patient 0" was a necessary narrative construction in order to write HIV as an outbreak narrative; "Patient 0" serves four narrative roles: he is a tangible target of who brought HIV to the US (when the reality is there were likely several entry points); his sexual practices make him someone with personal responsibility and stigma; he embodies both the public health dilemma, thus allowing for a focus on normalizing sexual behavior, and the "the malevolence of the virus" (233). Narratively, "Patient 0" represents a connection to a "dark continent," Africa; "the continent enters his body through the virus, which in turn crosses boundaries through his body" (237).

of HIV-positive people remain unknown to the Centers for Disease Control (compared with only 22 percent remaining unknown in Canada) (84). Smith and Agrawala determine that the demographic shift where HIV has gone from affecting gay men to "straight black women" is one where infection rates go from "visible to invisible," this invisibility a result of Black women historically being underrepresented in the US health-care system because they lack health insurance (86). Looking for, and analyzing, the writing of women living with HIV helps make this epidemic visible, and, in doing so, we find that the Cold War metaphors of invasion and containment become increasingly less important as the intersections of racial, class, and gender oppression take a heightened importance in the role of first-person narrators, whether fiction or memoir. The problem is not primarily an alien form of contagion but centuries of America-born discrimination itself.

We begin to find women in the US writing about HIV first in the form of fiction, with Sapphire's *Push* published in 1996 and gaining a resurgence in widespread readership following Tyler Perry's adaptation to the major motion picture *Precious* in 2009 and with Pearl Cleage's novel *What Looks Like Crazy on an Ordinary Day . . .* published in 1997 and gaining widespread readership when selected for Oprah's Book Club. While several memoirs had been written by people living with HIV in the US prior to 1995 (most notably, perhaps, Paul Monette's *Borrowed Time,* published in 1988 and tracing his own experience with HIV and the loss of his partner, Rog), few of those memoirs referenced cis-gendered women's experiences with the diagnosis. *Push* and *What Looks Like Crazy on an Ordinary Day . . .* were the first to trace the experience of Black women with HIV at a time when Black women were the fastest-growing HIV population. They also both address issues of family and intimate partner violence as well as reproduction and sexuality for heterosexual women, making them distinct contributions to HIV literature in the 1990s.

The first memoir we see written by a woman in the US living with HIV is Catherine Wyatt-Morley's *AIDS Memoir: Journal of an HIV-Positive Mother,* published by Kumarian Press, a small African American press, in 1997; in 2012 Wyatt-Morley published another memoir, *My Life with AIDS: From Tragedy to Triumph,* which shares many of the same details as her first memoir (now out of print) but in a different format. The first memoir is told primarily in the style of a journal, tracing her experience from her diagnosis after a hysterectomy and the later divorce from her husband (who contracted the virus through infidelity and then infected Wyatt-Morley), through her experience founding a HIV activist and support group for women. Throughout the memoir, Wyatt-Morley shares her experience as an African American mother of three and a factory worker, emphasizing how HIV diagnosis has complicated her experience as a single mother. She also includes photographs of herself and her children throughout, calling on readers to recognize her through her motherhood.

Paula Peterson also centralizes motherhood in her memoir, *Penitent, with Roses: An HIV+ Mother Reflects,* published in 2001. The book is marketed to a higher-literacy market. Peterson writes as a White middle-class married woman who discovers her HIV diagnosis years after initial infection, when she becomes ill following the birth of her son. Like Wyatt-Morley's, Peterson's positive status is discovered during routine gynecological medical care and presents a different set of medical concerns, distinct from the primarily cisgender male memoirs of the 1980s and 1990s. By situating their experiences of HIV diagnosis as part of their reproductive experience, both Peterson and Wyatt-Morley write against what Wald and Foertsch conceptualize as the construction of the HIV virus as alien by writing a virus as within, using their female-bodied experiences of gestation to queer and disrupt conceptualizations of self and other. While Wyatt-Morley includes family portraits to emphasize her role as a mother, Peterson emphasizes her motherhood through a closing letter written to her son. Motherhood, in both memoirs, becomes a key rhetorical strategy for narrative connection to readers.[6]

Regan Hoffman's memoir, *I Have Something to Tell You,* is the first by a woman living with HIV in the US that does not rely on rhetorics of motherhood. Publishing in 2009, Hoffman was already known to the HIV community as an editor of *POZ,* a magazine of HIV news and feature stories distributed free through AIDS service organizations. Hoffman writes of her surprise diagnosis as a wealthy young White woman—a strategy that perhaps emphasizes all people's vulnerability but that also works to distance her from women of color and gay men. However, she spends the second half of her memoir writing about HIV globally, situating herself and her intersectional privilege as part of a diverse, global, and vulnerable community.

Marvelyn Brown similarly situates herself as part of a global community in her book *The Naked Truth: Young, Beautiful, and (HIV) Positive,* published in 2008. Before publishing, Brown was also a known activist, appearing on shows like *America's Next Top Model* and telling her story in an MTV PSA as part of the *Greater Than AIDS* Campaign. Brown is the first memoirist I write about to come of age during the HIV crisis; as an African American teenager from Tennessee, she writes of the failures of abstinence-only education, the

---

6. For more on HIV and motherhood in Peterson and Wyatt-Morley, see my chapter in Michael Rembis's edited collection *Disabling Domesticity* (Palgrave Macmillan, 2016).

sacrifices her illness caused her to make as an athlete, and her future as a heterosexual woman who may want to become pregnant. Written twelve years after Wyatt-Morley's, Brown's memoir still reads, in part, like a public service campaign, citing statistics and prevention, continuing her public persona as a speaker and HIV educator. By framing herself in this way, Brown is able to brand herself as an HIV spokesperson, monetizing her own stigma within the political economy of stigma.

These were the memoirs written by women living with HIV in the US at the time of my first reading group. Since then, another memoir has been published—the first by a child born with the virus. Paige Rawl writes, in *Positive: Surviving My Bullies, Finding Hope, and Changing the World,* about her experience as a child and teenager with HIV, coming out to her classmates, and a lawsuit she files against her Indiana high school for failing to protect her against discrimination from both her peers and her school administration. Rawl writes about her relationship with her mother, who is also living with HIV, as her primary supportive relationship; the present absence in Rawl's memoir is any reference to her own sexuality and negotiations of sex while living with HIV, despite her being a college student at the time of writing. Like Brown, Rawl uses her memoir to situate herself and her HIV advocacy amid a conservative political landscape.

These women writers help us understand that HIV is not an individual impairment to be triumphed over; it is a complex interaction of institutions of power that have historically neglected and/or abused Black women. My argument here is not only that we gain a more complex understanding of how disability operates by incorporating HIV memoirs in our theories about disability life writing, but that previous theories about rejecting triumphant endings in light of a more nuanced understanding of disability identity are incorrect. In fact, while I locate HIV memoir precisely in Couser's formulations of autosomatography and the memoir boom, all memoirists formulate a triumphant ending for their narratives. Similar to what Anna Mollow argues in her analysis of Meri Nana-Ama Danquah's memoir *Willow Weep for Me,* these triumphant endings take on a different set of meanings for triumph, one that allows the reader to understand life writing itself as a continuation of HIV advocacy and activism within a neoliberal marketplace.[7]

---

7. For more on how Marvelyn Brown's memoir, in particular, unsettles notions of triumph within disability studies, please see my previous writing in *a/b: Journal of Autobiography Studies.*

Catharsis, Triumph, and Writer Motivation:
Insights from Reading Groups

It is an early spring day when Elizabeth and I meet for the last time to talk about her experience in my HIV reading group. Before we met, Elizabeth did not read much; in the privacy of a local AIDS service organization's conference room, I ask her whether anything has changed for her in the six months since we began meeting. Elizabeth discusses the combination of reading and group discussion as more helpful in understanding her HIV than her experience with doctors and support groups in the past five years: "It brought to light a lot of things I need to check out for myself. I think I'll always love autobiographies now" (3/14/2013). For Elizabeth, the memoirs did serve as an educational tool, but they also served to highlight barriers to her own medical care—leading Elizabeth, alongside other group members, to develop a sophisticated political consciousness. This same consciousness is not as apparent in my reading group of AIDS service workers, many of whom continue to read and reinforce tropes of pity and triumph through individualizing diagnostic practices. For example, in relation to reading the memoir of Marvelyn Brown, a young African American woman who contracts HIV as a teenager, the latter group members asserted that Brown's experience was one of bad parenting and needing to "find love," understanding her as a person to pity; this is in contrast to understanding Brown as responding to the failures of comprehensive sex education that helped her develop the political consciousness to become an HIV activist and public speaker. The barriers to Brown that led to her lack of understanding of HIV transmission were not discussed in the book group of AIDS service providers. Whereas for Elizabeth, Brown's book highlighted the failures of institutional systems of care and education, shedding light on her own experience, for some in my AIDS service worker group, Brown's book only highlighted individual failures.

In my initial interviews with AIDS service workers, my participants tended to address the question of author motivation as one that is therapeutic. As Marge, a patient peer advocate at a local ASO and a White woman in her sixties, told me in our first meeting:

> I think they need a way to get it out—writing it. I'm not sure they would even need people to read it after they wrote it. It's just not anonymous but people don't really know you, that kind of thing; it's a way to get it out there because it is good therapy to write. And I've learned a lot about how you feel in women's groups and mixed groups that I go to psychiatrically. How we aren't treating the whole body, and I care a lot about doing that. (3/13/2015)

Marge is my only research participant who is both living with HIV and working in the AIDS service industry. She is the participant in my group of AIDS service workers most hesitant to share her views on our readings initially, perhaps related to her different educational background (she does not have a college education), age difference (she is older than the other group members), and serostatus. Even so, her response that the motivation for writing is therapeutic aligns with the responses from other participants in this reading group. As Gretta, a social worker in the group, tells me, "I think it helps you to release it" (4/17/15). In response to my question about why one would write memoir about an illness or disability, Gretta reflects on her experience working with her sister to write about her sister's experience with domestic violence: "It was my sister's ability to really put it down on paper and read it and write it and then let go of it. [If you don't do this] it becomes murkier and murkier and then it seeps into the rest of you and then your personality and you aren't able to live" (4/17/2015). For Gretta, in analogizing the experience of illness or disability to the experience of domestic violence, she imagines the experience of HIV as having an oozing, horror-film quality; if the ooze is not contained on the paper, it has the potential to take control of one's whole life.

Others in the AIDS service worker reading group understand memoir as conveying a universal experience, eliding an understanding of how oppression and privilege operate to increase vulnerability for some. This, in turn, allows some to understand themselves as similar to those they read while ignoring the systemic and institutional oppression that shapes individual experience. As Adam, a psychiatrist in the local ASO, tells me, he reads memoir and autobiography to understand "the human experience": "My perception is that humans are very similar. So, I could learn a lot about what I could experience in the same experience" (3/17/2015). Adam speaks perhaps more explicitly about the need for this predictability; his expectation for universality in narrative—an expectation I address most explicitly in the following chapters—reinforces intersectional stigma and highlights precisely how expectations of universality create genre expectations that market to a White, middle-class, able-bodied consumer-citizen. For example, some members of the ASO reading group tired of reading about the experiences of women of color, a feeling they expressed as minority fatigue (and that I address in more detail in chapter 3). But this "minority fatigue" can only happen when there is a universal expectation of how the narrative should work; the fatigue happens with the presumed deviations from the universal.

Diana, a woman who has been doing HIV advocacy work since the beginning of the movement in 1982, diverges from the idea that one writes purely for therapeutic purposes, though she does emphasize that it is "cathartic" to tell your own story about illness. But of HIV memoirs, Diana tells me, "It is so life changing. It becomes you. And of course, if you work in health care, it is all life consuming" (3/13/15). Here, Diana speaks of the utility of the HIV memoir, first by serving as therapeutic tool for the writer; and second by sharing the specifics of an illness experience that are unique and thus serve as a tool for learning for HIV and AIDS service providers and/or the family members of those living with HIV. Unfortunately, for Diana and others in the AIDS service worker reading group, those living with HIV themselves are an afterthought in the population reading these memoirs.

Other members of this group do imagine a seropositive audience. Nick, who has the personal experience of having a cousin living with HIV, envisions most explicitly an audience of those living with HIV reading memoir about HIV, first by envisioning himself in the aftermath of the first few months of diagnosis: "So, I contract HIV, I am having a really hard time with it, the stigma is too much, so why not have a book, you know?" Notably, Nick is unable to envision himself as living with HIV throughout the entire scenario—the "I" of experiencing the stigma of HIV moves to the "they" of selecting the book from a bookstore shelf and "relating to" it: "They can go to a bookstore, go to a library, and pick a book up off the shelf and read it and really relate to it; this is how they got through it, you know?" (5/15/2015). The function of the memoir becomes one of finding a common experience through the particularities of shared stigma related to HIV.

After we read several memoirs together as a group, I returned to this question of "why write?" in my final one-on-one interviews. Through the process of reading together, and reading memoir, which was not his usual choice of reading, Adam expands his understanding of author motivation: "I think memoirs can do a lot to show people because you get to hear the personal experience of the author and how they interact with the world; it gives us a glimpse into privilege and things like that. In my case, I just wouldn't understand [some experiences] because I have privilege—other than being gay, which has reduced my privilege a great deal" (11/24/2015). Here, Adam talks about the utility of the memoir while not actually addressing the author's motivation; we can assume that the author may have the motivation of "showing people" the particularities of living with the stigma of HIV or disability; however, Adam continues to imagine a disembodied audience, never identifying the "them." This disembodied audience is a part of how the political economy of stigma works; the narrative circulates with an expectation of universal reception, obscuring how the narrative itself is shaped by systemic oppression and privilege, reinforcing the stigma of personal failure and the beneficence of medical practice.

When I asked my other participants whether they had read memoir during the course of their training and/or professionalization, all said no. I asked all members of this reading group whether they felt memoirs should be used as a more formal part of medical training; they all agreed that they should be, as a means of building empathy. Tony, a MA student in the sciences who joined the group partway through when he began his work as a test counselor, tells me, "Studies show that if you go from first-year medical school to fourth-year medical school, your empathy for the patient was really high the first year and by the time you hit the third year, that point is the lowest." He argues that "having memoirs and stuff will increase [empathy]—I don't think it will increase it 100 percent, but it will increase the empathy of it" (12/11/2015). When I asked my other participants whether they had read memoir in the course of their training and/or professionalization, all said no. I also asked whether reading memoir would be an important part of ongoing professionalization. All agreed that it would, although they emphasized repeatedly how much the memoirs would facilitate their personal collegial relationships, as opposed to their relationships with their clients. However, no one ever mentioned the idea of reading memoir alongside their clients in a book-group-type setting (though there are ongoing support groups that would enable this kind of sociality); only one participant said that he had recommended one of our books to a client. Those living with HIV remain invisible as a reading audience, even for those who work daily with people living with HIV. While I address in more detail what may account for this invisibility in later chapters, what I want to emphasize here is the invisibility itself, which in turn shapes my group's analysis of writing motivation being limited to therapy for oneself (the writer) and empathy (for the reader).

My reading group composed of women living with HIV had a different interpretation of why someone living with a chronic illness or disability might write and share their experience, as they shared in their first interviews with me. While they also suggested that some motivation might be therapeutic, they highlighted motivations of social change and social justice as well as more logistical financial concerns.

In my first set of one-on-one interviews with women living with HIV, it was a popular understanding that people wrote memoirs in order to break feelings of isolation; memoirs were written to connect with others who may be undergoing something similar. Elizabeth also thought it might be "self-therapeutic" for the person writing the book, emphasizing personal growth in the process of writing (7/24/2012), echoing what Diana expressed to the ASO worker reading group. Others, however, expressed motivations other than therapy. Judy was the most enthusiastic in our first interview when answering this question, eager to discuss how her interest in the group developed from her own goal of writing her autobiography (8/23/2012). When I asked more specifically about why she thinks other people write autobiography, she was self-reflective: "Well, my interest in it is writing an autobiography about my life is to be, uh, inspirational to other people, women and men and society. I want to leave an impact on others, and I want them to know that the choices that you make, and you don't have to go down that road, and try to avoid going down that path that I've traveled" (8/23/2012). Here, Judy switches from first person to second person, attributing agency to herself and then her reader. She also speaks of wanting to be inspirational while at the same time alluding to shame in her own experience and cautions her readers not to make the same choices.

In the six months of our reading and discussing memoir, Judy often calls our authors "inspiring" and cites inspiration as her motivation for reading. While Thomas Couser and other disability theorists have critiqued the emphasis on inspiration in disability memoir, I want to caution here that this inspiration Judy experiences may not be the same: Judy and my other research participants living with HIV find inspiration to address logistical medical concerns and larger social justice issues; this is distinct from the inspiration porn that Stella Young and others have addressed, because these women living with HIV are not objectifying disabled people for able-bodied benefit.

In our final interviews, after doing much of the same readings as the ASO worker group, all three participants responded to the question of why someone might write an autobiography in more depth. In my chapter opening, I discussed the role that memoir played for Elizabeth as a tool for education and self-advocacy. Elizabeth's response resonates with other group members. Judy found encouragement: "I was encouraged by the books because they led me to understand that I also can start writing. That a lot of women out there do not have the boldness to share their experience with HIV. And AIDS. And other illnesses. Any illness" (3/26/2013). Judy theorizes a connection between stigma and HIV and other illness; she also understands writing as a kind of activism. And, without provocation, she cites the production and circulation of memoir as a product:

> In so many ways, I don't think it has anything to do with "I can make some money." That too, but I think, you know, they want to speak out, be activists, share their stories, so they can get known or something like that. But I think

it goes farther than that. I mean, I think it is about speaking out and sharing their story so they can help a person who may be struggling as well, who is closed in, who feels like maybe they can't share. Got to be careful about sharing it to other people. (3/26/2013)

Here, Judy exhibits more confidence in discussing motivation for writing autobiography than in her first interview, theorizing both the economic benefits (though some of our memoirs came from small presses where economic benefits were likely negligible) and the activist work of destigmatization. And, finally, Judy ends her response with a note of caution, emphasizing that disclosure can be risky. This echoes the process that Judy underwent in writing her own story during our time in the group; when we first met, she was in the beginning phases of writing a testimonial to be shared with her church. By the time of our final interview, she had decided, after meeting with her pastor, not to share her experience. While she never disclosed to the group why, she did mention that she did not feel her writing itself, grammar and sentence construction, was where she wanted it to be, a realization that came, in part, from her first community college class.

In all my interviews about the role of autobiography in this first reading group, books never existed as a static entity but functioned as a dialogic tool for building relationships—with each other, with me as a researcher, and, in some cases, with their families. Elizabeth tells me of an exchange the books prompted with her daughter-in-law:

So, the last time you gave me all them books and I took them home she was like, "why you got all them books? I've never known you to read books," and I told her, I explained to her about me joining this women's book study club and that we were going to get all of these books and that it had a lot to do with, a lot of women having to find out their HIV status and stuff like that. I said, "You know, I'm really happy to be in this because, you know, for a long time I didn't tell you." She goes, "I know." I said, "This is like giving me a chance to solidify the whole thing of me going through this. Not only that, I am also going to be engaged with other women going through the same thing [. . .] This is really going to help me because I am not comfortable with disclosing to people." (2/7/2013)

The context of Elizabeth relating this interaction of disclosure with her daughter-in-law, not just disclosure but the disclosure of the pain in disclosure, comes sandwiched between the shared readings of Marvelyn Brown's memoir. Sometime after this discussion, but before Elizabeth had gotten around to it, Elizabeth's daughter-in-law read Brown's memoir herself. Elizabeth describes it to me this way:

> E: I just happened to pull it out and read the back of it [Brown's *Naked Truth*]. I set it down and started doing something. Well, my daughter-in-law picked it up and she read it. Read the whole thing.
>
> A: Really?!
>
> E: I was like, "Don't tell me about it! I gotta read it myself!"
>
> A: Don't give it away.
>
> E: Yah. She was like, "Ah, Mom, that's good. That's a really good book." I said, "Really?" She said, "Yah, you're going to really like it."

And indeed, Elizabeth did really enjoy the memoir, citing it as one of her favorites from our time together. The memoir works as a liaison between Elizabeth, her HIV, her daughter-in-law, and me. The book functions not just as a narrative where Elizabeth and her daughter-in-law relate to moments in the text (for instance, Elizabeth talks in detail of the similarity between Marvelyn and her sister and her own sibling experience) but also as a product, the memoirs themselves drawing attention with their paratextual elements (Elizabeth reading the back of the book, Elizabeth's daughter-in-law picking the book up absent-mindedly while visiting the apartment). This moment captures the mobility and circulation of memoir within a social network, disrupting the political economy of stigma which does not anticipate embodied readers that would read through their embodiment to develop a sophisticated political consciousness. Disclosing her serostatus is a means for Elizabeth to address oppression and privilege in her own life and in the community around her, destigmatizing HIV illness.

While attention to mobility and circulation is key to understanding life writing, life-writing theorists too often focus on life writing as a static entity, creating taxonomies that prescribe and limit our understandings of life writing. While current life-writing theorists understand the social construction of identity in life-writing practices, they do not theorize the practice of reading life writing. Many women living with HIV related to all the memoirs we read, whether they were about HIV or another chronic illness or disability, not because of the factual elements of the life story being told explicitly but because these factual elements highlighted similarities to and differences from their own experiences. The women living with HIV in my reading group never presumed to understand the memoirists' true experience but instead, as we see in later chapters, moved in and out of relating to authors and each other in a mobile, ever-changing way.

This ethical relation highlights the mobility of identification; a key site to analyze how mobile identification work is in the production of recognition in life writing, an investigation that emphasizes life writing as a product within neoliberalism. As my field research in this section has shown, identity matters in how one interprets an author's motivation to write about their experience with stigmatizing illness. Those readers who directly identified with the experience of living with HIV highlighted the material negotiations of the authors, while those without that experience understood the authors' motivations as therapeutic.

While scholars have provided important critiques of the common tropes of disability, including themes of horror, spiritual compensation, and triumph within the disability life writing that emerges during the memoir boom, few have actually addressed how women of color writing about disability may transform our understandings of these tropes (Couser 2009; Smith and Watson 2010; Mintz 2007). Judy, for instance, imagines the utility of her own life writing through inspiration, wanting to inspire others to avoid some of her own life paths that led her to contract HIV. When Couser laments that much of disability life writing does not include women of color, he is perhaps understanding disability too narrowly and missing conditions, such as HIV, that disproportionately impact communities of color. It is not just that women of color are writing HIV memoir but that when White women and class-privileged women write HIV memoir, they write in comparison to Blackness, as Peterson does, distancing herself from it, or in recognition of Blackness, as Hoffman does. This causes the women living with HIV to avoid these memoirs, finding them unrelatable. Writing about HIV, because HIV has disproportionately affected women of color in the US and women in the global South, is always with a visibility to racial oppression. Further, examining life writing about illness that is episodic, not static, and invisible broadens our representations of disability and allows for understanding how different groups of readers may relate to memoir in resistance to stigmatization.

In the next chapter, I read three HIV memoirs closely for their negotiation of material labor, highlighting how the memoir industry itself reinforces intersectional stigma. Two of these memoirs, Wyatt-Morley's *Journal of an HIV-Positive Mother* and Hoffman's *I Have Something to Tell You,* were selected by popular vote in both reading groups, providing me the opportunity to compare and contrast reader receptions. I analyze these reception in the next chapter to demonstrate how stigma circulates as a product for consumption by the neoliberal consumer-citizen.

CHAPTER 2

Writing Labor,
Writing Privilege in HIV Memoir

Hosting two different reading groups gave me the opportunity to explore disparate reading receptions, particularly in instances when group members chose the same texts from their lists of options; the selection process itself highlights overlaps in reading interests among the group members living with HIV and those working as an AIDS service provider. Both reading groups chose to read the Hoffman and the Wyatt-Morley memoirs. Participants living with HIV in my first reading group overwhelmingly disliked Hoffman's memoir, citing class difference as rendering the memoir unreadable—this despite their optimism going in to the memoir because they are all avid readers of POZ, the HIV magazine where Hoffman was an editor. Referenced in my introduction, this is the book about which Elizabeth said "I couldn't get past her and her damn horse!" For participants who were AIDS service workers, Hoffman's memoir was an overwhelming favorite. This distinction between reader receptions highlights the mobility of reader reception and the importance of labor and class negotiations in the construction of reader–writer relationships in relation to disability and medicine; this is what creates the political economy of stigma, disenfranchising those with chronic disabling conditions by situating their conditions as an effect of personal failure and professionally rewarding medical providers for procuring patient narratives: the more oppressed the patient, the higher the reward.

Previously disability life writing has been understood as individual productions—static entities—as opposed to mobile products that invite disparate receptions from readers. How readers consume life narratives about illness and disability is deeply dependent on their own relationships to intersectional privilege and their relationships to illness and disability itself. Indeed, we cannot understand tropes of triumph or pity without looking at narrative as a circulating product within a neoliberal market. In what follows, I provide a close reading of Wyatt-Morley and Hoffman, as well as a third memoir, Paula Peterson's *Penitent, with Roses,* to investigate how intersectional privilege affects readership and circulation.

HIV and the Welfare Queen: The Emergence of HIV Memoir in Relation to Welfare Reform

In the memoir *Journal of an HIV-Positive Mother,* paid labor plays a central role in how Catherine Wyatt-Morley conveys the daily experience of living with HIV in the mid-1990s (1994–96). The central arc of the memoir is Wyatt-Morley's reimagining of the role of work in her life, moving from working-class factory employee to community leader and head of a media start-up, rejecting the stigma of the welfare queen. At the same time, she contrasts her own productivity with that of her husband's increasing inability to work, investing in an ableist logic of productivity and deservedness to stake a claim on citizenship. By centering paid labor, in conjunction with her consistent emphasis on her motherhood, Wyatt-Morley writes against a "welfare queen" representation, which took on heightened significance at the time of her writing due to Clinton's 1996 Welfare Reform Act (Hancock 1–10). The welfare queen representation,[1] which conveys poor Black women as hyperfertile and lazy, leads to what Hancock terms "the politics of disgust" (1–25). As Hancock explains, in welfare politics, democratic attention is perverted into "ideological justification for a specific policy," which separates welfare recipients from other "worthy" Americans (3). I argue that this is key for thinking about who gets empathetic attention in terms of HIV. Stereotypes and moral judgments are bestowed upon groups subject to government welfare policy (15–17). Exposure to public identities (based on stereotypes and moral judgments) causes citizens to devalue some citizens' claims to resources and results in the public's alienation from political participation (18). By emphasizing her negotiation of

---

1. There is much important work done in Black feminist studies on the welfare queen stereotype, including but not limited to Hortense Spillers, "Mama's Baby, Papa's Maybe: An American Grammar Book," *Diacritics* vol. 17, no. 2, 1987, pp. 64–81; Patricia Hill Collins, *Black Feminist Thought: Knowledge, Consciousness and the Politics of Empowerment* (Routledge, 1990); and Cathy J. Cohen, "Punks, Bulldaggers, and Welfare Queens: The Radical Potential of Queer Politics?" *GLQ: A Journal of Lesbian and Gay Studies* vol. 3, no. 4, 1997, pp. 437–65.

workplace accommodations in the plant following her initial HIV diagnosis, her unpaid labor creating a media start-up, and her work as an increasingly single mother of three school-aged children, Wyatt-Morley effectively writes against the welfare queen stereotype, subverting this politics of disgust and asserting herself into a democratic space, by focusing on her negotiations of labor in the context of HIV stigma and HIV-related illness.

Wyatt-Morley, writing in a journal format, first discusses her negotiations of labor and illness when, after a three-month sick leave following surgery and subsequent HIV diagnosis, she returns to work. Here, we see Wyatt-Morley negotiating disability accommodations within her physically demanding factory job; she is also negotiating the need to work to support her family (her husband, also recently diagnosed with HIV, is having much more difficulty than she and is often unable to maintain hours). In mid-July 1994, she writes, "I'm back at work but I'm really not feeling well enough to be back. Bev [Wyatt-Morley's good friend] wanted me to stay out longer, but I had to come back because my pay has been at 60 percent since June. The company has not changed since March; neither have its people. I was not put on a job, so I sat in the cafeteria waiting for a supervisor to find a job within my restrictions" (Wyatt-Morley 1997, 17). Her emphasis on working while not feeling well, and the lack of paid work available to her based on physical restrictions, counter stereotypes of laziness.

While Wyatt-Morley is focused on working to support her family, a few journal entries later she discusses how she begins a support group for women with HIV, WORTH (18). WORTH develops from a support group to an advocacy organization, centering "the needs of working mothers who are sick, women as heads of households, dental care, gynecological issues, and the aloneness we all share" (24). Notably, material, economic concerns are listed before medical and emotional needs. In writing about her volunteer work, Wyatt-Morley emphasizes her ability to participate in a labor force if her current paid labor were less physically demanding. During the time Wyatt-Morley is founding WORTH, her factory job is unable to provide appropriate accommodations; it takes two months for her supervisor to find her a "temporary placement" (27–28). This juxtaposition between the factory work and accommodations, and her HIV coordinating and volunteer work, is a consistent narrative technique throughout the memoir; often both are discussed in the same journal entries.

Activating workplace accommodations creates a series of vulnerabilities for Wyatt-Morley, from having to out herself to HR in the early days of the ADA, when it was less effective than intended,[2] to creating a reason

---

2. Ruth Colker writes about the first ten years of the ADA, the period when Wyatt-Morley is seeking accommodations, as being less than effective for plaintiffs. In 2008 Congress

for interpersonal interactions with authority figures that would lead to abuse. Wyatt-Morley recounts her experiences of sexual harassment by her supervisor, who calls her at home when she takes sick leave (28, 34). Amid this harassment, Wyatt-Morley begins to attend national HIV conferences with her group. "I'd like to work in the fight against HIV and AIDS," Wyatt-Morley writes in November 1994. "I want God's words to come from my mouth as I speak against the lack of education that has occurred among our youth or for universal healthcare for every American. We need to be educated" (35–36). By connecting her activism to educating youth in particular, Wyatt-Morley indirectly connects her labor with motherhood. She is also consistently demonstrating her increased professionalization in the emerging field of HIV care and advocacy. For example, on January 12, 1995, Wyatt-Morley attends a conference in Kentucky, detailing her own growing knowledge of clinical trials and HIV medication while educating her readers (43). Throughout the book, Wyatt-Morley recounts what she learns at these conferences, demonstrating her knowledge and educating her readers (43–45, 47–49, 85–87, 92). The book itself becomes a part of her educational advocacy.

As Wyatt-Morley becomes increasingly professionalized through her volunteer work, her wage work continues to present problems in relation to her disability and her gender (the power relations that lead to sexual harassment). Directly following her recounting of the Kentucky conference, Wyatt-Morley writes a short entry about her supervisor's harassment: "The supervisor from the plant continues to call my home. When I'm not at work due to illness, taking a vacation, or whatever reason, he calls. His continued advances toward me have become unbearable" (45). After an extended sick leave following a diagnosis of a seizure disorder, Wyatt-Morley returns to work, again experiencing a lack of accommodations: "He [her supervisor] looked at my restrictions and laughed. I will be in this area a month before I can be moved" (74).

> I am sitting in the cafeteria at the plant, where some of the restricted people sit who have no job. I listen to them tell one another the latest news about who was put out and why. It feels humiliating to be put on display surrounded by others with options. I think about what it's like to be here, and what other people with HIV must be going through when their employers have no workplace policy to protect against HIV discrimination. It scares me. Leadership, both union and nonunion, has done nothing to place individuals with disabilities. Forcing disabled employees out appears to be the

---

passed the ADA Amendments Act, which would help alleviate some of these early difficulties that ran counter to the ADA's intention. See Colker, *The Disability Pendulum*, and Feldblum, Barry, and Benfer, "The ADA Amendments Act of 2008."

company's way of handling sickness, workplace injuries, and terminal illness. (101)

Here, Wyatt-Morley understands herself as part of a group with disability, a
group of individuals "without options" because they cannot participate in the
labor of the plant. As such, she understands the need for linking HIV and disability advocacy in the workplace.

Wyatt-Morley recognizes herself simultaneously as an empowered advocate through her media start-up and as a vulnerable worker through her
position at the plant; HIV is the "driving force" for both realities. As Wyatt-
Morley's HIV-related conditions cause more physical problems, such as car-
pal tunnel and peripheral neuropathy, she begins a women-and-HIV media
project. In doing so, Wyatt-Morley again educates her readers, walking them
through the process of writing grants, finding producers, conducting interviews, and promoting the project (52, 57, 75, 76. 90–91): "HIV is the driving
force behind me doing this video. I would be working at the plant and going
on with my life if Tim and I were not infected with this virus" (54). Development of the video project weaves itself through the book, often directly pre-
ceding her medical updates:

> *March 28, 1995.* Things with the video are moving slowly. There's so much to
> learn. I told Tim that I spend more than ten hours a day doing or thinking
> of things to incorporate into it.
>
> Went to the doctor today. Bev said I was
> doing great. I told her that I feel good,
> other than my hands. (55)

Here, Wyatt-Morley not only juxtaposes her video project with her physical
disability that causes her problems with working for wage labor at the plant;
she also counts her hours, writing against any stereotypes of laziness. Count-
ing her hours becomes a way to claim value as a citizen in a neoliberal nation
where productivity is a central tenet of personhood. It also marks a habit of
blue-collar wage work that stands in contrast to the often-salaried white-collar
work with which she is getting acquainted through her activism.

Another way to establish her value is to contrast her own physical condition sharply with that of her husband, who is increasingly unable to work
entirely: "Tim got up this morning, got dressed, kissed me goodbye, went
downstairs, sat on the couch, and could not move. When he doesn't go to
work, I can bet something's wrong" (61). When Wyatt-Morley has her first

HIV-related seizure, she recounts the experience to her readers by first writing about how "June 22 was like any other day" and that she was on her way "to pick up a letter recommending me to serve on the Tennessee HIV/AIDS Community Prevention Planning Group" (70). We learn these details before learning of the seizure. The seizures do not interfere with Wyatt-Morley's ability to travel and participate in national HIV/AIDS conferences (102–3, 116–17). Thus, Wyatt-Morley values her own productivity through an ableist logic that emphasizes her husband's deteriorating physicality and inability to work. She needs to characterize her husband this way in order to create an effective literary foil and cement her own claims to citizenship.

Wyatt-Morley eventually sees the need to merge her volunteer advocacy with paid work: "Well, I have given it great thought and I think it is time for my work life and private mission to become one. I can no longer live in 'if.' It's time 'if' got a life. My work with the video has taken me many places" (117). Wyatt-Morley comes out as HIV-positive at work (141), takes her video to film festivals, tells her own story in media outlets (140–82), and procures a book contract for the memoir we are reading (168). Wyatt-Morley centers her material negotiations with HIV in order to write against the welfare queen stereotype and to undermine the politics of disgust. As Wyatt-Morley becomes increasingly disabled in the context of her paid work, she becomes a powerful HIV advocate, experiencing a change in her own understandings of power.

By writing against the politics of disgust and the welfare queen stereotype, Wyatt-Morley also invests in the ableist logic of productivity to stake a claim on citizenship; these seemingly contradictory logics are easily accommodated within the political economy of stigma, which can valorize disability as productive and inspirational when it is indeed productive and stigmatize those same conditions when they fail to morally rehabilitate the individual into a neoliberal market. Here, the medical industrial complex and individual self-advocacy that emphasizes the importance of institutional fairness and a moderate redistribution of resources to productive workers become the solution to multigenerational systemic oppression; meanwhile, the systemic inadequacies of the medical industrial complex and workplace accommodations are obscured through individual failure and bad luck.

The Worthy/Unworthy Citizen in HIV Memoir

Paula Peterson also centers her experience as a mother and HIV advocate in her memoir, *Penitent, with Roses: An HIV+ Mother Reflects*. Whereas Wyatt-

Morley writes against the politics of disgust by centering her negotiations of paid labor and HIV, while also investing an ableist logic of productivity, Paula Peterson, a White, married Jewish mother, reinforces the worthy/unworthy citizenship divide differently. Not only is there a notable absence of economic and labor negotiations, but the ways in which Peterson continually emphasizes her White, married, heterosexual subjectivity, in contrast to women of color and poor women whom she meets in her search for community after her HIV diagnosis, reifies the divide between worthy and unworthy. Additionally, Peterson's memoir is marketed as a more literary text than Wyatt-Morley's, published in conjunction with the Breadloaf Writer's Conference / University of New England Press. With her constant references to graduate school and writing as "art" (not work), and her own writerly identity, Peterson distances herself from the self-conscious activist texts of Wyatt-Morley, whose publisher, Kumarian Press, is marketed toward African Americans and centered on social justice work. While Wyatt-Morley writes about procuring her book contract, and the economic opportunity the contract opens for herself and her family, Peterson never mentions the material negotiations of writing a book or even pursuing an MFA in creative writing. In short, Peterson's memoir is one of "art," not labor or advocacy, and her HIV is isolated from other social justice concerns.

In her memoir, Peterson writes about herself as an advocate, but her book itself is not part of the advocacy, an important distinction from Wyatt-Morley. Peterson is not trying to educate a broad audience about HIV through this writing. The book, written as a series of freestanding literary essays, is intended to be an artistic exploration of contagion, motherhood, and contemporary relationships within the experience of HIV. In the opening chapter, when Peterson recounts her caesarean section, she writes herself against any stereotype of hyperfertility:

> In my twenties, I harbored a romantic notion that I was "barren." This may have been reinforced by the fact that, as a young girl, too thin and too athletic, I often went six months or more without having a period; I had also been on the Pill for many years and had been told by a doctor that the hormonal interference might make conception a lengthier process. And as a writer, I nursed a conviction, quite legitimate, that any fertility that I possessed would be manifested through my art, not my body. (5)

Although Peterson does not deny promiscuity here, with reference to taking birth control, she does write herself as "responsible," concerned with having children before monogamy, while also potentially as so disciplined (athletic, thin) that she is actually the opposite of lazy and hyperfertile. Establishing herself as disciplined and responsible, she also establishes herself as an artist, writing not to make ends meet but because of some inner drive, some innate sense of self.

As Peterson recounts the process of her diagnosis following the birth of her son, she again resists stigma: "I told myself I had the advantage of having contracted a very public and political disease that instantly conferred martyrdom on its sufferers" (28). Although Peterson is not as explicit as Wyatt-Morley in the period of her diagnosis, we can understand, based on the timeline Peterson does provide (referencing her probably contracting the disease in 1985 and having had it for ten years by the time she was diagnosed), that she is experiencing her diagnosis at the same historical moment as Wyatt-Morley. But geographically, not just being on the West Coast but experiencing HIV in proximity to White, upper-class activism, Peterson has a less stigmatized association with her diagnosis. She writes: "You could not have a more fashionable disease. In San Francisco, at least, the stigma was not as pronounced. Your civil rights were indisputable" (28). At the same time that she understands her HIV in proximity to Whiteness, she also does not feel a part of the HIV community: "It was not 'my' disease. [. . .] I did not know anybody else like myself—white, Jewish, middle-class, college-educated, and HIV-positive. I tried turning it all upside down and thinking about it in a different way. This was a more successful tactic. It was funny but I turned out to be exotic after all" (29). Here, Peterson, in one of many iterations, emphasizes her Whiteness and class privilege, as well as her education and religious/ethnic heritage.

In a paradox, Peterson does not feel the stark stigma related to HIV because of fifteen years of destigmatization work of White male activists in San Francisco; she also understands her HIV racially. It makes her "exotic," an Other, and in mid-1990s multiculturalism, this is desirable. Yet, she establishes herself as an anomaly in the HIV community (and, by extension, not deserving of HIV).

In the chapter "Who We Are," in which Peterson rehearses statistics related to women with HIV, she again emphasizes her own Whiteness. "Being a white woman with HIV in the United States, a white Jewish woman at that, puts me in a unique position. It's a lonely place to be. I discovered after my diagnosis that I had very little community, especially if I wanted to scrape together a community out of women who fit my demographic specifications. I soon abandoned that idea and began looking for women, any women" (71). Here, Peterson does not tell us why race, class, gender, and religion are important in her relationship to HIV, assuming that the reader will just understand this. These distinctions are not about relationships to power and social justice that make salient communities grouped along race, class, and gender lines. While these distinctions are *explicitly* demographic and descriptive, reading closely reveals that Peterson *implicitly* believes that race and class are an immediate window into worthiness between her and other HIV-positive people. Her Whiteness and class privilege become her claim to reader empathy.

Peterson goes on to describe a retreat for women living with HIV, writing almost as if an anthropologist, observing and recounting participants' life stories while giving an hour-by-hour description of the retreat's activities (71–106). She provides physical details that are coded with racial and class judgment and understands herself as a member of the HIV community only in relationship to White workshop organizers. The first two women Peterson describes, as she does throughout the chapter, with a sense of detached observation:

> Two women in wheelchairs introduce themselves: Joanne, square, chinless, with tiny eyes and a flat forehead. A thug's face. She had long sparse reddish hair that an attendant, standing behind her, is combing and re-braiding. The other, Martina, is younger, smaller, and softer, with brown moist eyes that seem filmed over. Next to her chair, the paraphernalia of the oxygen deprived—tank, tubing, carrying case. Both are chain smokers, dropping their ashes on the sidewalk, directing their unflinching gaze into the middle-distance. Joanne converses with me but Martina is not as accessible. (73)

Here, Peterson describes the physical details of appearance, without describing facial expressions. For Peterson, details are focused on the body but not the person. Through her observation, Peterson judges these participants negatively, describing one as having a "thug's face" and both as chain-smokers, despite their reliance on oxygen. These women, in Peterson's short reflection, are irresponsible, unhealthy, and dependent on others for care. At their meal later in the day, Peterson attributes an animal-like paranoia to Joanne and Martina: "they eat solemnly, glancing from side to side, as if they fear someone is going to cheat them of their portion" (77). Peterson also describes the food: "black-eyes peas, cornbread, meatloaf. Several of the Black women whoop with joy" (77). By describing both the food and the other participants as having childlike or animal-like qualities, and by beginning the chapter by emphasizing her own White, middle-class subjectivity, Peterson sets herself apart from the participants. In contrast to the participants, Peterson describes their workshop leader, Eve, who is living with HIV, positively: "Hazel eyes and seamless ivory skin. A voice that is always in excellent tune. Hers is an authentic beauty: she draws from a deep well of grace within her" (78). Again,

Peterson focuses on the physical details of Eve, attributing a personality trait through the physical descriptions of Whiteness. It is within this context that Peterson understands herself as part of a community: "But I notice the shadows in her cheeks. The slight sunkenness. The oversized sweater probably hides the thickened waist. These are the signs by which we know one another" (78). By providing detached observations of women on the retreat, Peterson functions as a reporter or anthropologist. This juxtaposition between herself and the retreat participants reinforces a deserving/undeserving binary of HIV subjectivity.

In a chapter titled "Working the Line," Peterson analogizes volunteering at a San Francisco HIV hotline to factory work. Unlike descriptions of factory work, however, Peterson begins her chapter thus: "I settle myself into my booth with a cup of coffee, after schmoozing with my neighbor" (105); here, the workplace has a sense of relaxation and comfort, not the bustling pace of an assembly line. This suggests that Peterson has a white-collar relationship to work, making Peterson appear oblivious to the majority of the world's population living with HIV. Peterson's "working the line" stands in sharp contrast to Wyatt-Morley's work at the plant.

She conveys stories of hotline callers, presenting herself as knowledgeable, expert: "I force myself to ask, my heart beating rapidly, whether she has nursed her children. 'Of course, miss,' she says proudly. 'Every single one for a year.' She does not seem to understand that the virus can be transmitted from mother to child through breast milk." In the process of presenting to the reader her own knowledge and training as a hotline volunteer, she conveys her caller as ignorant, a "young African woman" with a "pleasant sing-song accent" (114–15). The power hierarchy, cultural differences in understandings of disease, access to barrier protection, and attention to poverty never enter into Peterson's analysis. In fact, she ends her chapter coupling this simplicity with one of her few insights into her work life: "Fondly, I imagine that thousands of men are now using condoms correctly because of my advice. ('Never use an oil-based lubricant. Roll out the air bubbles. And for God's sake, check the expiration date.') That thousands of women will now buy condoms themselves and insist their partners wear them [. . .] These airy fantasies sustain me for the week between my shifts" (123). Here, Peterson reinforces her own hotline expertise by emphasizing that she is volunteering, one four-hour shift a week. In between shifts, she "fantasizes" about her own White savior persona, a superficial aggrandizement of her individuality. Although she is equipped to offer advice about condoms, she does not provide the reader a deeper analysis of health inequalities and economic negotiations for people living with HIV. Instead, Peterson contrasts herself with a "young African woman" in a way that reinforces stereotypes of African ignorance and White superiority as opposed to highlighting her own experience, detailed in her first two chapters, of nursing her son without knowledge of her HIV. Peterson is not interested in understanding herself as part of a community with her callers.

Peterson reinforces this deserving/undeserving divide when she discusses the financial negotiations of a group trip to advocate of HIV policy in Washington, DC, the only time she mentions finances in relation to HIV:

> All of us have been allotted a small sum of money for this trip and most of us feel the amount has been generous. Several of the women, however, have spent all of their money and have nothing left to get them from the airport to their homes. One woman has been begging money from a few other women in the group, myself included. We suspect she may be an alcoholic. (136)

In a narrative where economic negotiations are notably absent (How does Peterson make a living? What does her husband do? How does she access / pay for her medications?), her attention to the financial details of this trip seems superfluous. It does nothing to illuminate why women on the trip would need an allowance in the first place (Why are many women with HIV living in low socioeconomic conditions? Are they on a fixed income or Social Security? Do their medication side effects cause them to lose hourly wages, as in Wyatt-Morley's case?). Instead, readers get Peterson's explanation of alcoholism (read: irresponsibility) in contrast to Peterson's own sense of gratitude—the allowance, for Peterson, is "generous." Peterson does not address the social inequities between herself and the other women in her "activist" group. Peterson's advocacy, what she calls her activism, stops at her own Whiteness and class privilege. Her story about HIV is a story that reinforces White privilege and undermines HIV social justice work.

In the final chapter, before Peterson begins her closing letter to her son, she writes about her work on Capitol Hill, reinforcing her ambivalence around social justice and enforcing her understanding of HIV in isolation from other inequalities. This work is a microcosm for the book's project itself:

> At the age of thirty-nine, on the brink of middle-age, I set out to save the world. I am an activist. Tentatively, I mouth these words, and by the third or fourth time I have spoken this sentence, it begins to seem credible. [. . .] I have good reason to doubt myself because for most of my life, I have been indifferent to world affairs. It is only for the last few years I have developed a political conscience. Once, in graduate school, I got dragged into a march

against apartheid, but it was only because I was on my way to the library and the marchers happened to cross my path and one of them was my advisor, who pulled me in, and I felt for the sake of my academic career, I couldn't refuse. (124)

For Peterson, genocide is simply one of many "world affairs" that does not enter her "political conscience"; apartheid is in the same category as voting rarely in local elections. Notably, while ACT UP activists framed the Reagan-era response to HIV as a form of genocide, Peterson's writing is tone deaf to the history of HIV activism and framing. While it could be argued that HIV awakened Peterson's political consciousness, she does not demonstrate an investment in social justice work anywhere else in the text. In fact, she writes of her legislative speech as a "performance"—"a story about my story" (133)—again framing writing as art as opposed to an economic negotiation that addresses power inequalities.

As she discusses her work in HIV advocacy on Capitol Hill, she again reinforces this deserving/undeserving divide by emphasizing her own White-ness in order to gain political attention for HIV: "Our biggest enemy, what we have really come to fight, is this attitude that AIDS is a disease that happens to *other* people" (130). Again, Peterson reinforces this deserving/undeserving divide by emphasizing her own Whiteness in order to gain political attention for HIV. Because she is not an "other," HIV warrants legislative attention.

HIV Memoir as White Privilege

Regan Hoffman's memoir, published by Atria Books in 2009, an imprint of the mainstream press Simon and Schuster, is the most recently published of the three memoirs I discuss in this chapter; in contrast to Peterson, Hoffman addresses race and class privilege in both national and international contexts, expanding on her experience as editor of *POZ*, an HIV magazine dissemi-nated through AIDS service organizations and other medical-social networks. Hoffman's HIV diagnosis, like Wyatt-Morley's and Peterson's, occurs in the mid-1990s; at the time of her diagnosis, Hoffman briefly took AZT and was given one year to live. Within two years, she was seeing an HIV specialist and taking new protease inhibitors, pharmaceuticals that greatly increased life expectancy for people with HIV and decreased medication side effects. Hoffman's intersecting privilege, particularly economic and social, is central to how she situates her experience with HIV.

Hoffman opens her memoir with attention to class detail, such as when she mentions her first marriage falling apart because of different lifestyle expectations: "Andrew wanted to play golf and have me wait for him in a crisply-pleated tennis skirt at the country club's nineteenth hole" (11). Raised in Princeton, New Jersey, and a graduate of the Trinity College, Hoffman, in recounting her moment of diagnosis, writes: "As long as I did the right thing, my instructors taught me, I would be safe" (19). She contrasts her own life with the *Jerry Springer* show unfolding before her in the doctor's office, as she waits for the results of her blood work: "I was thinking of how glad I was to have been born in a world far, far away from *Jerry Springer*'s guests" (19). These class signifiers are written into the first third of the memoir as descriptive detail of her background. Her reflection on class, however, moves from descriptive to analytical as her experience with HIV progresses. Her first move toward the analytical occurs in the closing line of the chapter discussing her diagnosis:

> On the way out of the doctor's office, they asked me to pay my bill. They should not do this. Perhaps they bill you on the spot because they worry you will go home and blow your brains out. In case you're wondering, they charge you $250 to tell you, you are dying. (24)

This attention to the cost of medical treatment foreshadows the economic negotiations that become central to her national and global analysis of HIV. That this is the closing line in the chapter about her diagnosis emphasizes the neoliberal experience of health care in the US.

After her diagnosis, which happened in the year following her first divorce, while she was freelancing and "training horses to help pay the bills" (38), Hoffman agonized over telling her parents and needing to move back in with her mother for financial support: "I had faltered and made a mistake that was going to cost us all a lot of money, social disgrace, agony, and probably my life" (45). Hoffman emphasizes her economic negotiations here alongside the social and embodied implications of HIV. While her financial negotiations of HIV remain important in the text, Hoffman is also aware of the social implications of HIV within her upper-class community:

> To everyone around me, I seemed healthy, affluent, well-educated and privileged. I'd gone to private school. I had a degree from Trinity College in Hartford, Connecticut, and post-graduation, had run with a fast, wealthy, international crowd in New York City [. . .] I worked with CBS News and other top advertising agencies. [. . .] Which made it particularly hard to

admit that I derailed my chances of success by getting a terminal disease. (64)

Hoffman simultaneously recognizes her social and professional loss due to HIV while emphasizing her economic privilege in the face of a nurse who refuses to draw her blood. "But I wondered: What happens to HIV-positive people who can't find the right kind of support? Do they ever speak to their families again? Do they ever go back to the doctor?" (66). Hoffman consistently recognizes her access to the most advanced AIDS doctors in New York City and Philadelphia (91). This section of the narrative, where Hoffman begins to recognize the intersection of her own privilege and oppression through HIV, is the beginning of her politicization of privilege, found in the rest of the text.

Hoffman begins to work training horses at a neighboring farm, writing: "All the reasons I couldn't justify for taking a job with low pay and high physical risk vanished in the face of HIV" (94). While Hoffman does not recount how she is paying for medical insurance, she is clear about living simply, either with her mother or in a friend's barn. She also mentions no need to put money into a 401(k), a tenet of middle-class financial stability. Once Hoffman realized how effective the new medications were, and developed the expectation that she would live to a "normal life expectancy," she decided to return to editing and writing, working for a lifestyle magazine (105). While doing this, Hoffman also began writing an anonymous column for *POZ* about her experience as a woman living with HIV (126). Eventually, she was asked to apply for the position of editor (131):

> I had already achieved one of my career goals—I had become Editor-in-Chief of *New Jersey Life*. But as much as I loved the magazine and working with Cheryl, I had always dreamed of being a war correspondent, or writing stories about life—and death. Working for POZ would not make me a war correspondent. But it would take me back to earlier days, when I wanted to have an impact on people's thinking by doing groundbreaking stories on volatile and taboo subjects—and by writing about life and death. (132)

Unlike Peterson, who writes of her political engagement as a complete turn of character, Hoffman understands her HIV as enabling her to return to some of her earlier goals—this time with an unexpected twist of reporting about HIV. Analogizing HIV to war allows Hoffman the rhetoric to conceptualize the life and death struggles of HIV while not making too simplistic of a comparison. HIV is not a violent battleground. This is an important distinction, writing at a time when people living with HIV have access to major pharmaceutical interventions and when the US, at the time of her publication, had been at war in Afghanistan and Iraq for more than five years. While Peterson simplistically equates anti-apartheid activism with her short speech on Capitol Hill about HIV, she erases key sociopolitical differences and valorizes her White privilege in the process. Hoffman's analogy, by contrast, politicizes HIV while resisting the conflation of war with infection or disease.

Once offered, Hoffman hesitates about taking the job at *POZ*, worried that she doesn't correctly "represent" the majority of people living with HIV. Unlike Peterson, who continually addresses how her being White, middle-class, and educated makes her an HIV anomaly, Hoffman locates herself in a larger, global picture of HIV:

> When I scrolled through the data in 2006, I was shocked to discover that women comprised 47 percent of all infected people worldwide. In the United States, nearly a third of all people living with HIV were women. I looked at the numbers again and again, feeling a strange mix of emotions: on the one hand, I was glad to discover I wasn't a freak; on the other hand, I was horrified that awareness and prevention efforts had failed so miserably around the globe that the numbers of people infected with a preventable disease were exploding. (135)

At this point, roughly halfway through Hoffman's narrative, we again see a shift. Hoffman begins to write about HIV at a global level, locating herself here as a part of that epidemic, as opposed to an anomaly. Through HIV, and the socioeconomic negotiations that led her to work at *POZ*, Hoffman is able to address the global economic divides and politicize preventable disease: "It was a welcome change to write about such meaty things as congressmen blocking bills that would secure access to care for all HIV-positive people, the latest HIV treatments, and the travel ban that prevents HIV-positive people from entering the United States" (138). In her global analysis of HIV, Hoffman does not locate HIV solely in the "Third World" and or in poverty; she implicates the US as a key offender of social justice for people living with HIV. She writes, "Many of our most brilliant and tenacious HIV activists were dead, or tired, and I didn't see overwhelming evidence that what was left of the old guard was nurturing future generations of AIDS activists. If more wasn't done, AIDS was going to continue its deadly spread—at a frightening exponential rate" (145–46).

In this same chapter, in stark contrast to Peterson's perspective, Hoffman questions the utility of her HIV disclosure to the public at large, questioning the conflation of disclosure with activism (146–48). Simultaneously, Hoffman does write about how taking the job at *POZ* gave her a freedom and a sense of relief that accompanies her disclosure. This distinction between disclosure as socially and psychically beneficial (166–80) and disclosure as activism is key in Hoffman's use of her own story in politicizing HIV/AIDS and enabling a new generation of activists.

Through her work at *POZ,* Hoffman interacts with many international activists, both at conferences and in traveling abroad to research. When speaking with a group of women from Malawi, Hoffman is clear about the economic negotiations of working with HIV in the US: "I told them about my job at *POZ* and how lucky I am to be able to afford health insurance, which covered the costs of my treatment. But I also explained that I lived in fear of a day when, because of HIV, I'd get too sick to be able to work, and therefore wouldn't be able to afford health insurance and my own care" (194). Because the US connects access to comprehensive health insurance to employment, the global HIV community can understand people with HIV in the US as marginalized. As Hoffman writes, "The balance between my health and my ability to work to make enough money to pay for my life-saving treatment was a fragile one" (194). While the material negotiations of people with HIV are different in the US from those of people with HIV in Malawi, as Hoffman recognizes, the lack of comprehensive health care in the US creates unstable life conditions for people with HIV/AIDS. Hoffman, in her travel and research, balances delicately between holding the US accountable for its own inadequate HIV resources and policy and recognizing the economic destitution that greatly reduces the life span of people living with HIV in the global South.

In her final chapters, Hoffman writes about government neglect of people with HIV in relation to the New Orleans flood (drawing a human rights analogy at first but also connecting the neglect to the literal bodies of people living with HIV in the city; 215–19); the prison industrial complex (and the policies and procedures around how meds are distributed and made intolerable; 219–20); international access to condoms and, in the US as well as globally, women's lack of empowerment to ask partners to use condoms (221–23); HIV orphans in Southeast Asia (228–37); and funding for the Ryan White HIV/AIDS Program (253). Taking on the voice of HIV activist, Hoffman brings material negotiations for people with HIV to the forefront: "Taking away someone's dignity by treating them as if their life is not worth living is bad enough; being so afraid of someone that you take away their housing and medical care is unforgivable. And it happens every day, all over the world, to people living with HIV" (234). While Hoffman consistently brings attention to her research and puts HIV in a global context, she also does not allow readers to see her as a disembodied Western charitable savior; she is always embodied, her HIV is always present, and she reminds readers that what she is doing is work:

> After lunch, while starting to make my way home to the hotel, I realized I felt unwell. My body was feeling the effects of being under stress, in sweltering countries, constantly surrounded by strangers, always having to be "on." I'd had trouble eating; my medicines take away my appetite and I couldn't find any of my comfort foods in this land of lychees and chicken boiled in hot oil. So far the only familiar food I found was cornflakes. (244)

Even with her body as uncomfortable as it is, she goes to her meetings with activists and policymakers; attends dinners and conferences, taking notes for her *POZ* publications; and uses her own HIV story as a point of connection between activists. She centers her own survival, this idea that she might die before significant steps are made in HIV policy and in biomedical research, which detracts from an image that she is selfless: "I was driven in part by fear, that there was too little being done to fight the global pandemic, that too many will get sick and die, that I will die [. . .] So I ate a bowl of cornflakes back at the hotel and sucked it up" (244). By centering her body in her activism and by using her own race and class privilege to draw attention to HIV locally (she writes about speaking at a country club in the town where she grew up) and internationally, she politicizes HIV, and the material negotiations of HIV, in a global context.

All three women in this chapter write about their experience with HIV diagnosis in a time before protease inhibitors, when an HIV diagnosis was a death sentence. They also all write about themselves as new medication is discovered and they must now negotiate a longer life expectancy in the face of HIV stigma. As cisgender women, they are minorities among the visible HIV community. In order to stake a claim on citizenship, they engage reader empathy by sharing intimate personal details alongside larger ruminations on self-worth and care. Wyatt-Morley, an African American mother of three from Tennessee, does so by writing against the politics of disgust and the welfare queen stereotype, adopting an ableist logic of emphasizing her own productivity and motherhood. Peterson emphasizes her own Whiteness in order to situate herself as an HIV anomaly to gain sympathies for herself as an individual artist, distinct from many of the African American women she frames as irresponsible and animal-like in her memoir. Hoffman shares the narrative of her HIV diagnosis while complicating her place as both privileged and oppressed and situating her responsibility to the global HIV community as a relatively privileged White American. While all three women stake a claim on citizenship for those with HIV, they do so by at times reinforcing racist, ableist, sexist, homophobic, or classist stereotypes; at other times, these stereotypes are fractured. All three narratives circulate within the political economy of stigma, mediating author–reader relationships that can reinforce tropes of pity and triumph while also producing, in the case of Wyatt-Morley and Hoffman, valuable HIV educational tools that can disrupt medical disenfranchisement for those living with HIV. These memoirs provide useful medical information while demonstrating how one can advocate for oneself with doctors and policymakers. The political economy of stigma, like any neoliberal economy, embraces these messy contradictions.

In the next section, "The Privilege of Privacy," I analyze how life narratives are interpreted and circulated among medical professionals. In the section's first chapter, I look more closely at the reader responses of AIDS service workers, analyzing a pattern of reception that I call *diagnostic reading*.

PART II

THE PRIVILEGE OF PRIVACY

CHAPTER 3

Diagnostic Reading and the Limits of Disability Memoir

It is a chilly day in late September; the semester is in full swing, and I have just arrived at the ASO staff lunchroom for my fourth reading-group meeting with AIDS service workers. As I am taking off my coat and simultaneously arranging the chicken kebab and falafel I have brought for the group's lunch, group participants start to stream in. We all talk casually about the weather, and I am feeling grateful that our initial first meetings are over; we fall into a friendly, comfortable conversation about work and teaching. Without prompting, one participant, while balanceing a paper plate of lentil salad and chicken on top of his copy of this week's book, *Willow Weep for Me*, tells me that he is not sure whether this has to do with a conference he was at just the week before or with the book itself, but that he is "feeling minority fatigue" (9/29/2015).

I am unclear what that means but realize that in this moment before the rest of the group arrives, we are talking queer White person to queer White person. "What about me and my perspective as a White gay man?" he says (9/29/2015). I pause, wondering whether I should respond as I would to a student in my disability memoir class, reminding him of the importance of intersectionality in our discussion of the lived experiences of people with HIV, probing him for a close passage reading on the spot; as I pause, I know that I need to respond as a "researcher": my goal is not to persuade a particular understanding of the text at hand but to figure out where his own understanding comes from. Before I am able to respond to this participant, others filter into the room, asking me what I think of Meri Nana-Ama Danquah's memoir of depression and citizenship as a Black immigrant in the 1990s.

We are all falling into friendly banter with one another; I am understood as a member of their community and our conversations are opening up, becoming more candid. I am researcher–friend–fellow activist. I tell them this: that I will share with them at the end of our reading group session why each book makes the list of options but that what is important to me now is finding out their perspectives. As I turn the tape recorder on and settle into my seat, asking someone in the group to volunteer a synopsis of the book (our ritual beginning each month), I am wondering about this experience of "minority fatigue" and how this will resonate, affect our conversations, as the group moves forward. I am wondering how many others in the group feel similarly. And I am thinking about the women in my first group: how can their experiences with persistent daily oppressions be understood by their HIV practitioners if their practitioners are too "minority fatigued"? How tiresome is this oppression, and for whom?

In this chapter, I explore the dynamics of my ASO worker reading group, capturing the group's receptions to each book we read together in order to unveil patterns of reading; what I find in this analysis is a pattern of reception I call *diagnostic reading* that leads to a limited interpretation of the lived experience of people with HIV. Whose stories get heard is not simply about listening closely and reading closely but about cultures of reception that move beyond a medical model of selfhood. If, as I have been arguing, the political economy of stigma operates through mediating relationships between authors and readers in life writing, then we have to understand that no reader-receiver is immune to this mediation. How a book is marketed, in addition to how an author writes about her own relationship to writing and income, affects the interpretations of the value of the narrative for the reading audience (as we saw in my last chapter); medical practitioners, in particular, run the risk of reinforcing stigma in how they interpret their jobs as medical providers. The economy of relation produced through the production of stigma affects not only how a person living with HIV is afforded medical care but also how their stories themselves are interpreted. Through the political economy of stigma, a person living with HIV is always already a subject to be diagnosed.

ASO Workers and Diagnostic Reading

The group members I worked with were all colleagues at a local AIDS service organization; they included psychiatric nurses, social workers, doctors, and intake test counselors. All of the reading group participants had a politicized understanding of HIV because of their own relationship to the illness and/or their relationship within the LBGTQ community. Those ASO workers who did not tend to have this politicized commitment did not sign up for the group.[1] All members had an opportunity to vote on the titles they wanted to read, selected from two lists—one of HIV memoirs written by women in the US, the other a list of popular disability memoirs written by women in the US (see Appendix A). After initial one-on-one interviews, we met monthly for our reading group, extending the group from six months to eight months when they expressed interest in continuing to meet.

Reading disability and HIV memoirs with members of my ASO worker reading group unveiled a trend in reception that I am calling diagnostic reading. Through diagnostic reading, members of my ASO worker reading group continued to find narrative meaning through medical models of diagnosis; the participants consistently linked patterns of behavior and the internal disclosures of memoirists to patterns of psychiatric illness. This reinforces Julie Elman's model of rehabilitative citizenship, which encourages the proliferation of diagnostic media (from television shows to WebMD) in order to reinforce personal responsibility for health and wellness and to create corporate profits (172–75). Building on Elman's interventions, we can understand how this model of rehabilitative citizenship relates to the political economy of stigma, which produces a set of relations between medical providers, patient-consumers, and readers that stigmatizes those with chronic illness through tropes of personal responsibility and rewards medical practitioners for circulating individual narratives of disability sans (much) systemic analysis of oppression. By producing this set of relations, the political economy of stigma upholds the authority of the medical industrial complex, rehabilitating it in the eyes of the public despite widespread critiques of the MIC's fiscal and physical exploitation. In doing so, the political economy of stigma enacts rehabilitative citizenship through producing a diagnostic reading practice among medical practitioners.

The diagnostic reading of my ASO reading group led to a limited interpretation of memoirists' experiences and often negated the transformative activist potential of reading and writing memoir itself. Instead, their readings reinforced the larger interests of AIDS stakeholders (such as pharmaceutical companies) promoting pharmaceutical interventions over the downward distribution of resources to accommodate housing, food, and living expenses.

---

1. See the introduction for more about how I reached this conclusion based on my recruitment strategies.

This move of valuing pharmaceutical intervention over a larger HIV safety net, which was fought for and sustained for more than forty years (by some of the readers at the table), is an example of the larger move in HIV policy toward what HIV scholar Celeste Watkins-Hayes calls the "test-and-treat revolution" (178–203). Understood through the political economy of stigma, diagnostic reading enacts a form of rehabilitative citizenship for and through the medical industrial complex, reinforcing personal responsibility for HIV that values pharmaceutical intervention over broad systemic change.

This trend of diagnostic reading among ASO workers developed over the course of our time together; in the beginning, diagnostic reading was subtle, using a diagnostic term like *manic* to describe a memoirist's action, but by the time our group was reading our final memoir, its diagnostic reading was prominent, with some members choosing plot points such as a memoirist moving across the country as diagnostic evidence of bipolar disorder. Some diagnostic reading observations from the last few books we read together even called individual participants to reassess their readings of the first few memoirs we'd read together. This tendency to read diagnostically exemplifies what disability literary theorist Michael Bérubé warns against when he writes, "Disability studies need not and should not predicate its existence as a practice of criticism by reading a literary text in one hand and the DSM-5 in the other" (20); diagnosis does not "solve" a text (20). In extending Bérubé's thinking, I understand reading diagnostically not just as psychiatrically diagnosing characters and/or authors but as understanding characters and/or authors as singular entities that can be better understood through medical expertise. This reading practice can superficially include a recognition of oppressive social structures but does so only to descriptively contextualize an individual's sociopolitical circumstances; it does not, as Olivia Banner argues, allow us to "read for structures" (26–27 *Vulnerable Constitutions*).

The first book we read together was Marvelyn Brown's *The Naked Truth: Young, Beautiful, and (HIV) Positive,* a contemporary memoir of a young Black woman from Tennessee who acquires HIV as a teenager and goes on to become an HIV activist and public speaker (appearing for young audiences on venues for MTV and on the *Tyra Banks Show*). Since this is the first book we read together, the group was perhaps a bit more formal than they would be as our time went on, being careful to find positive attributes in the book. Even so, much of the group discussion revolved around "diagnosing" problems that led to Brown's exposure to HIV; for the group, Brown was disabled from the start.

It is important that this is the first book we read together and our first book group discussion, because while there was a tendency to read diagnostically in these early discussions, there was also movement to read empathetically, group members finding commonalities between themselves and the memoirists. This tendency to find commonality would dissipate over our time together. Diana, a long-term HIV activist and social worker, begins by summarizing the book this way:

> This is a very young, very young African American girl, who gets HIV, she is not the standard that people think, she is not promiscuous, she had sex with someone she loved, they used condoms, one time they didn't, they thought that was a commitment from him, but he turned out to be gay—or a downlow or just positive or—I think he's on the down low. And this is her struggle with being poor, low self-esteem, stigmatization that was terrible, and coming out above it but the struggle was immense and now she is, ah, well known and polished spokesperson for testing and prevention and care.

Note Diana's emphasis on Brown's age and "self-esteem," her personal conduct ("not promiscuous"). Her perception seems to be shared by the group; another participant echoes Diana's observation about Brown's self-esteem and adds that Brown "agoniz[es] over her boyfriend all the time." I have written elsewhere about the way Brown highlights her own ignorance as a result of a Bush-era policies against comprehensive sex education (Day 2013), but rather than understand Brown as responding to institutionalized structures of oppression, the group reads Brown's experience as one of individualized, even pathologized, struggle, highlighting her "low self-esteem" and what they read as an "obsession" with finding and keeping a boyfriend (6/8/2015).

Immediately the group connects Brown's story to that of their patients, contrasting the important generational differences between those diagnosed before 1996 and those diagnosed afterward:

> DIANA: What it reminded me of was our patients. You know? At first, I thought this was going to be some trite story of some young woman who overcomes adversity. Well, it wasn't. It was a lot of adversity. And it was a lot of stigma. It was like our patients, because they don't just overcome, they struggle, struggle, struggle and some of them make the best of it and do something with their lives and some of them stay in that struggle.
>
> NICK: Like we were saying yesterday about our patients, you know, some of them are elderly and they thought they would be dead by now, so they didn't have their midlife crisis. They didn't do the things they wanted to or should have done or whatever. And this is different. When she was diagnosed she was saying how the doctor was pissing her off and annoy-

ing her because he was like "Are you okay? Don't hurt yourself" and she was like "Just tell me what I need to do to get better," which is so different than I think it was in the beginning because there was no hope. In the early, early days.

This process of diagnosing Brown leads the group to pity her; Diana expresses this when Brown, after her diagnosis, uninhibitedly shares her experience with HIV: "And then she regretted it because everyone treated her so horribly. Poor thing. She didn't even know there was going to be a big shame factor to it" (6/8/2015). While the group shares this pity of Brown, two group members also relate to her. Gretta begins by discussing parallels with her own upbringing:

GRETTA: I get that. I had a mother that was exactly like her mom.
DIANA: She loved you, but she always put you down?
GRETTA: I don't know if she loved me. [laughter]
DIANA: Does now.
GRETTA: Okay, yes, I had a mother who had a very hard time expressing her love. But had a very easy time expressing how you dissatisfied her.
DIANA: Oh man, that's tough. That's tough.
NICK: My parents were super critical but also super loving. So, like, I never doubted their love for me. But they were so critical. So, when I was reading it, I was seeing parallels too, you know? But I mean I definitely have seen progression but like, in anybody's life, you take two steps forward, you are going to have to take two steps back until. . .
DIANA: She certainly did, didn't she? (6/8/2015)

Since Gretta and Nick are the two youngest members of the group, it is not as surprising to me that they might find connections to Brown with her cultural references to high school in the early 2000s (connections I share). What does make me pause as a researcher is their willingness to share, in our first meeting, past histories of trauma that allow them to relate to Brown, despite they themselves being seronegative. Even though Nick is vague in sharing exactly what his experiences are in this moment, later he relates to feelings of suicidality and despair:

Right. Um. And then realizing, well what is that going to solve almost. I mean, for someone who literally has been in that position it, um [pause] I know from my experiences like what is that goin' to solve? And I feel like she picked that out and realized this wasn't going to fix anything and I think, at one point didn't she say that would satisfy her mother or something like that? You know what I mean? Like those thoughts. And how when she got her diagnosis, it wasn't "okay, I'm going to die from this, what can we do." So that was really telling to me. Where, at first when she was in the hospital, she was like "this is my out. You know I am done. I don't have to be here anymore." But then it totally changed when the doctor said, "you have HIV." You know what I mean? So, I don't know. (6/8/2015)

As our meeting goes on, other members of the group continue to diagnose Brown; this happens particularly along generational divides. Adam says, "Before she ever got HIV she had low self-esteem. She was just beaten down" (6/8/2015). Diana follows up with another kind of diagnostic reading: "The things we learn about people with HIV, getting HIV, they are promiscuous but that comes from wanting to find unconditional love. And often they have been sexually abused as children and that gives them an unclear sense of their bodies and boundaries. And then raised in poverty and having no real father figure and no real mother figure that was loving, her father was absent, her mother was demeaning, I mean, you would be struggling for love all over!" (6/8/2015). Diana weaves her general experience with clients together with Brown's story, finding roots for pathology in personal trauma but avoiding a more politicized understanding of the extended Black family and generational poverty that Black feminist scholars have highlighted since before the Combahee River Collective Statement.[2] This may suggest that preparation for AIDS service workers should include an understanding of Black feminist thought just as importantly as it does (or should) include a history of the AIDS epidemic itself.

Our reading group met once a month, and I alternated HIV memoirs with other disability memoirs, memoirs often read in disability studies classes. The second book we read together was Lucy Grealy's *Autobiography of a Face*; Grealy writes about her experience with childhood cancer in the 1970s, which led to significant facial disfigurement and a complex relationship with plastic reconstructive surgery and pain management. The group struggled with this memoir. Gretta and Nick refused to read more than a few chapters because,

---

2. For example, see Barbara Smith, *The Combahee River Collective Statement: Black Feminist Organizing in the Seventies and Eighties*, Freedom Organizing Series 1 (Kitchen Table: Women of Color Press, 1986), and Patricia Hill Collins, *Black Feminist Thought: Knowledge, Consciousness, and the Politics of Empowerment* (Routledge, 2002).

after googling Grealy and finding out that she'd died from a drug overdose, they found the memoir unpalatable:[3]

> GRETTA: I like people that get over their issues and become a part of society and make it better. Not people that just hate society. And say "well they're all stupid." And that's what I felt like she was. And I didn't make it very far, I didn't even make it to the first chapter because I just decided the book where everything else that could possibly happen in the world is more important than me reading this book. (8/11/2015)

For Gretta and other members of the reading group, Grealy's inability to overcome her addiction in real life made the book "pointless" to read; these group members did not feel that a story was worth telling if there was not a triumphant lesson in the end.

Adam and Diana, in comparison, continued to read the book diagnostically, analyzing Grealy's relationship with her mother. The conversation organically led to a comparison of Grealy and Brown; the group questioned the role of autobiography as the genre in Grealy's book and decided that because Grealy is college-educated, she has a more intellectual approach to her life story whereas Brown's is more "behavioral"; I worry that this interpretation is supported by (subconscious) racist views of White people as intellectually superior to Black people. Gretta told the group, "I did not feel like it was written as an autobiography or if it was, I didn't like the tone of it" because "there were words that, I mean, I could figure out what they meant, but they weren't common words that I would use" (8/11/2015). Earlier in the conversation, Diana and Adam had made similar observations about Grealy's "intellectualism"; in the following passage:

> DIANA: She was so intellectual about things. She didn't talk about—it was about figuring out, looking for reason in pain, looking for enlightenment. And don't we all do this? I'm here in this moment, this will be the light and the truth, and I will follow this for my life to guide myself, and she would say, she would find it and say that only lasts for a second. And isn't that the truth? We are always looking in what we do a meaning in life and she was constantly, she needed to find meaning for the shit she

---

3. In her discussion of Grealy's memoir and Anne Patchett's *Afterward*, Rebecca Garden (2010) discusses how Grealy's overdose affects her reception, making a distinction for readers between the author and the authorial persona. Garden also identifies the market coercion to have a good patient narrative, one that Grealy's ending attempts to comply with but, following her death, greatly disrupts.

was going through, nobody else were going through this. And even 'til the day she died.

When I asked whether they thought they might be interpreting the intellectualizing they detected in Grealy's memoir as snobbishness, Gretta agreed: "I mean, yah, if you are going to label it an autobiography, it's got to be something about you as a person."

> GRETTA: If the title was different, and it was something about, you know, autobiography of a culture, or something like that, maybe it would be more, be able to read it more under a different understanding. But if you are going to say that it is your autobiography and it—
> MARGE: She calls it an autobiography of a face [emphasizing "a"] not her.
> A: Right. It's not "my" face. Well, what if you pretended it had a different title, would that help you?
> GRETTA: Maybe. If there were pictures of what she actually looked like. [laughing]
> A: On the back there is an author photo.
> DIANA: She doesn't look too bad.
> MARGE: She doesn't look disfigured to me there.

Significantly, the group goes on to "take back" many of their positive observations of Brown's book the month before. Regardless, they continue to understand the two women as psychiatrically disabled. The statement made reflects larger cultural conversations about pity and disability as well as racism and oppression. That Marvelyn Brown's experience is understood as fatiguing reflects not only the reality that her experience of sexism, racism, and poverty is marginalized in the larger discourse of HIV memoir, and thus notable to comment on in this manner, but also a feeling of frustration or hopelessness in our culture's progress in eradicating these systems of oppression. Minority fatigue is one discourse through which the political economy of stigma operates.

The third book we read together was Regan Hoffman's *I've Got Something to Tell You*; Hoffman is a White upper-class woman who acquires HIV and goes on to become an HIV advocate and editor of *POZ*, a popular HIV magazine funded by pharmaceutical companies. As I mentioned in chapter 2, this book was unreadable to the women in my first group, who were all living with HIV, primarily because her class status made Hoffman someone to whom it was difficult to relate; in contrast, my ASO worker group all voted this book as one of their top from our time together.

ADAM: So, when I looked at all three books, it was very interesting, I thought the three books that we read so far were primarily in a different domain. So, the first book it's all behavior: I did this I did this I did this I did this. The second book was all intellectual: I thought this, I thought this, I thought this.

NICK: You're right.

ADAM: This book actually made me cry. It was like "oh." It's like that doesn't usually happen with books with me [nodding around the table]. But she, it was a pretty emotional book, how it was written.

NICK: I think we all said that, that we cried. (9/8/2015).

Of all six books we read together as a group, this is the only book the group responded to with this kind of emotion; many group members related Hoffman's experience "coming out" as HIV-positive to their own experience as coming out as gay or lesbian. The group wrestled with the politics of disclosure: when disclosure is politically necessary; when it is ethically necessary; and when it is no one's business at all. Because Hoffman works as an HIV advocate, much of our group conversation revolved around the group's own experiences at work. In this way, they refrained from a purely diagnostic reading of Hoffman's book and were able to find similarities between her experiences with HIV and their own experiences with other kinds of stigma, as well as with their own work. Even so, they wanted more from Hoffman in relation to her medical diagnosis. They agreed that they want Hoffman to give more medical details and more details about her sexual practice in order to share with her readers practical, educational knowledge.

DIANA: I would like to hear more about sex. [laughter] Because obviously it's important.

ADAM: Of course!

GRETTA: I just mean she talks about sex and she talks about these are taboo topics and these are topics no one wants to talk about and they want me to talk about sex and then she never talks about how, like, this diseased body and then she moves from that to having sex with people.

ADAM: It's only the subtitle, "I have something to tell you," and you rarely got to sex.

GRETTA: Was the sex weird? I don't know. Maybe it was earth-shattering sex.

NICK: And I don't think her point in the book was to, was to, to talk so much about the sex so much as it was about her disclosing throughout her career.

DIANA: But I think a lot of people who are going to read this book who are positive would want to know how sex works. That's the thing. How does it work with a partner? Nobody seems to know until they get into that situation because they don't tell anybody and then they don't have sex.

NICK: Right. Well, I thought it was kind of important that if the people accepted her and understood. Like, I assumed she had sex with Jody. She said at one point, "Well, we went to bed" or something.

DIANA: Well yah!

NICK: So, my mind—

DIANA: But how did they accept condoms?

NICK: Right.

DIANA: I mean, people want to know, people who want to read that book really want to know how you have sex with somebody positive if you haven't done it for a while.

The assumption here is that the story is valuable because it can serve as an educational tool and that the education should have a practical application. This stands in contrast to the reaction to the previous passage, where the group was moved to tears—responding emotionally but not necessarily with an eye to practical application. The political economy of stigma, through which this group is responding to Hoffman's memoir, is capable of encompassing these seemingly contradictory responses, increasing the impact of the memoir on the seronegative audience. In reading Hoffman, the moments when the group could relate were moments when she spoke of her work as an HIV activist; when the group fell back into a more diagnostic reading, however, the value of the book was criticized as not being sufficiently educational. There was a consistent call for more medical detail.

The most significant practice of diagnostic reading came in our fourth meeting, when the group read Meri Nana-Ama Danquah's memoir *Willow Weep for Me*, published in 1998, which captures the experience of a Black immigrant woman with depression. I opened this chapter with Adam's reaction to Danquah's memoir as causing him "minority fatigue"; what I found in our discussion of Danquah is that the group's overwhelmingly negative response to the memoir was an effect of their practice of diagnostic reading:

ADAM: Um, I was really frustrated by the book when I first started reading it. It was like "ugh" something was wrong, it was chaotic, it didn't feel right, I'm reading it and I go "what's going on?" 'Cause I went into the book thinking I am going to read a book about a Black woman who is depressed and as I read along, I go, no, I am reading a wonderful story of someone who has been misdiagnosed. She is bipolar disorder.

DIANA: Yup.

ADAM: She is not depressed. I go, "oh my god, that's why it is so hard to get into the book" because the criteria for depression—she's bipolar! She has posttraumatic stress and nobody in the book addressed these issues.

A: So you came away thinking "she's just misdiagnosed."

ADAM: She is! [rounds of agreement]

A: Oh! Everybody thought that!

ADAM: I can pull out the book and show ya. She has elevation, she has high directed behavior at times, then she falls into depression, then she has impulsive—she goes out west, east and west, east and west.

DIANA: Uh-huh.

ADAM: She has volatile relationships I mean just ch ch ch [making check marks with his fingers in his palm]. Click off multiple criteria for bipolar; she's got it. (9/29/2015)

By the time I was having this conversation with our reading group, they had been talking with each other about *Willow*, something I certainly anticipated would happen when I created my methodology. What seems apparent to me is that Adam's perspective influences the group's reading, perhaps because he is considered more knowledgeable about psychiatric illness (as the head of the mental health component of their clinic's services); since many of the other group members are also trained as social workers, in systems of psychiatric diagnosis, it is also possible that they would draw these conclusions on their own. What is interesting is that because of illness, Gretta missed this meeting; in our final interview, Gretta told me that *Willow* was one of her favorite books from our time together because she could relate to both Danquah's trauma and her depression. Had Gretta been at this meeting, I wonder how the conversation might have been different, knowing her perspective.

What is striking about Adam's reading of Danquah's impulsive behavior is that many of us coming from histories of trauma, coming from socioeconomically depressed households, do not find moving across the country to live with relatives to be impulsive; we find it necessary for survival. What may be interpreted by someone as diagnosable impulsive behavior may be interpreted by others as uncanny survival skills. Tony, the only person of color in the group, and who arrived a little late to this lunch meeting, had this perspective:

I think it's really good. I think it's a good take on depression, especially for someone who is going through it. I actually really like the fact that they talked about seasonal affective disorder in it as well. Not a lot of people discuss that when you talk about depression, you talk about medications, you talk about what's going on in life, like, seasonal affective disorder, in a nutshell, part of that spectrum. So, I think it is a good thing that she discussed it in that regard. I felt like I was actually there with the author when she was talking about how she hated her husband; with the postpartum depression, when she talked about how she hated the child and everything like that, I thought I was actually in the book, when she was discussing this. (9/29/2015)

For Tony, the impulsive behavior is not on his radar; instead, he is appreciative of the disclosures of depression and the "realness" of her experience. Toward the end of our discussion, the group wanted to know my own perspective on Danquah's psychiatric illness; the diagnosis was important.

> MARGE: What do you think about our idea that she is bipolar and not depressed? Did you hear that before?
> A: Um, I'll tell you the truth; it doesn't matter to me.
> ADAM: [laughs]
> A: The diagnosis doesn't matter to me.
> MARGE: It matters to her if she's ever going to be normal.
> A: Sure. If she's ever going to be normal; but what is interesting to me is the, how she negotiates with medical practitioners, how she negotiates with her family, how she feels about her own experience. (9/29/2015)

The group is a little concerned at this point that I do not have the "right" priorities (as a disability studies scholar, I am much more interested in denormalizing normalizing rhetoric). This interaction may be a turning point in our relationship as peer activists because, as they go on to say, for them diagnosis is of the utmost importance because it affects the kind of treatment and medication they prescribe. What is interesting to me in this moment is that the group overwhelmingly decides that they do not like the book because of what they understand as Danquah's misdiagnosis; they ascribe the book's ending, which is not a "triumphant" ending in a more commercial sense, to this lack of correct diagnosis, as opposed to other structural barriers related to racism, sexism, and xenophobia that Danquah experiences.[4] In fact, for

---

4. For a complicated discussion of Danquah's invocation of triumph, see Anna Mollow, "'When Black Women Start Going on Prozac.'" In my own discussion of Marvelyn Brown's

Adam, the book is unpalatable because of what he understands as Danquah's anti-medical-establishment view.

> ADAM: But we have to understand that she, this book has an anti-medication, anti-treatment being she is Christian Science. That is from the very beginning; her childhood exposure to church is Christian Science and then we have this "no pills, no pills, no pills, I don't take pills for headaches, I don't take pills"—so we have a whole Christian religious, Christian Science religious theme going through this book that if you are not careful, you will miss it all together.
>
> DIANA: It's there.
>
> MARGE: You're right.
>
> ADAM: The other thing.
>
> DIANA: I didn't think about the Christian Scientist though I really paid attention to that in the beginning. I forgot; I thought it was just being African Ghanaian culture.
>
> ADAM: No, it was. Because she attacked Prozac right in the beginning, and you go—whoa! Because that drug was targeted by the Christian Scientists to destroy that.

While others in the group missed Danquah's Christian Scientist upbringing, Adam's reading brings about a subtle anger from the group. I am surprised by this reaction; in my teaching of this book and in my first reading group, I found readers to be overwhelmingly positive toward Danquah's memoir, finding it candid and relatable. The ASO worker group's practice of diagnostic reading inspired frustration and anger in response to Danquah's text. How does this relate to the minority fatigue that Adam confided in me at the beginning of lunch? I wonder how much this fatigue comes from Danquah's experience with multiple systems of oppression and how much of it comes from seeing an institution you are invested in—the medical industrial complex—fail over and over again?

We can connect this possibility that Adam's fatigue is symptomatic of the challenge to his professional expertise and power; this is similar to other narrative practices within medicine. For example, Lisa Diedrich argues in her analysis of HIV narratives written by doctors such as Rafael Campo and Abraham Verghese that "some doctors' narratives not only enact a possibility of *an-other medicine,* in which doctors are infected and affected by their patients,

---

memoir, I also invoke Mollow's interpretations of triumph as it relates to Black women with disability.

but also inscribe, or reinscribe, the reality of the same old medicine, in which doctors are omnipotent and omniscient figures and patients are the objects on which the doctor's power/knowledge is enacted" (2007, xxii). In extending Diedrich's ideas, we can see how power/knowledge is also enacted in the reading of patient narratives, not just in the writing about their own care work with people living with HIV.

The last two books we read together demonstrate how medicine itself came to be understood as a target of criticism by memoirists. The fifth book we read together was Catherine Wyatt-Morley's *Journal of an HIV-Positive Mother,* the first memoir written by a woman living with HIV in the US. Whereas this book was one of the favorites for my first group, my ASO worker group disliked it because of its style and age; as I mentioned in chapter 2, many group members did not feel that the book remained relevant, because it was so "historical." One way the group discussed its so-called irrelevancy pertained to the pharmaceutical and medical interventions that Wyatt-Morley explains to her readers; the group felt that because it was outdated, the book was not giving medicine a fair representation.

The final book we read together was Audre Lorde's *The Cancer Journals* (1980), which many of the members were eager to read because they had heard of Audre Lorde as a lesbian activist and there were decontextualized passages of her writing posted on the walls in their workplace. While a few group members found Lorde's writing too difficult to read, others (Adam and Diana) rated Lorde's book a favorite; despite its being the oldest memoir we read together as a group, Diana found it politically relevant:

DIANA: I think the basic message—I mean, maybe because I am older, I'm worried about cancer and death, maybe because I worked at a cancer center for so many years, maybe because I lost friends to cancer, maybe because I'm a feminist, I don't know, every couple of pages, I'm like "and that!" [mimicking underlining in her book] You know? Just off, it made me, the thing is this is written in 1978, just put somebody there, [reading] "In this disastrous time when little girls are still being stitched shut [. . .] in order to be more attractive to men" that means the medications, the cream, stuff that's got all this shit in it that causes cancer [reading] "When 12 year old black boys are shot down [. . .]." This is 1978. What little twelve-year old boy just got, Tamir Rice.

MARGE: A year ago.

DIANA: So all this stuff is still going on, if she, I'm going to go on, do you mind? [referencing a scrawl of page numbers and notes written in the front pages]

MARGE: Nope. [laughter all round]
NICK: Preach! (11/24/2015)

Even in the context of this recognition of Lorde as "political," none of the other memoirists were recognized as such. Because Diana was so eager to begin our conversation with the political connections to today's Black Lives Matter movement, and the group's overall enthusiasm for reading Lorde because she is well-known lesbian feminist activist, they refrained from some of the diagnostic reading practices that had become so prominent in our previous few meetings. As Adam said, with a somewhat ambiguous tone, "I just found it to be quite political"; Diana responded enthusiastically between bites of falafel, "Of course it is! That's who she is!" (11/24/2015).

> DIANA: The bottom line of this, I think, is that if you look at death and you face it, and she did, and she did for fourteen years, you shouldn't be afraid of anything. And what women, particularly oppressed people, are afraid of is their own voice, and speaking up to power, or to speaking their thoughts or feelings or telling the world they are fucked or whatever, and she, that's what she always wanted to do as a radical Black feminist lesbian mother, how she defined herself, she wanted to talk about those things with her sisters and with the world, and it's fearful and it's scary to stand up and do those things. So what she says, once she figured out she was going to die, is there is nothing to lose, so why not say anything she wants and not keep it to herself? So, I thought "that is such a good message!" I mean, I think all of us are activists in one way or another in our hearts, but it's hard to stand in that corner, and it's hard to confront that cop and blah blah and it's hard to confront the system. (11/24/2015)

Certainly, the structure of *The Cancer Journals* lends itself to political critique more readily than do the other memoirs, which are linear and in chapter form, whereas Lorde writes *The Cancer Journals* in two essays and one series of journal excerpts. For Diana, the political nature of Lorde's writing reinforced her own identity as a political activist; perhaps this is most significant for Diana because she was working in the local feminist movements at the time of Lorde's writing. For Diana, the message of Lorde's work was resistance.

In the group discussion, however, Lorde's perspective on her own healthcare needed to be tempered:

ADAM: It is great for what it is, but it is not a perspective on the world. She has a very clear political view and she does a beautiful job writing about it and if you go in with more than that, then you are going to be misled. With her view of society, it's like "Really?" I'm just coming like this was kind of narrow, politically narrow feminist.

DIANA: I don't think she pretends to be anything else!

NICK: Right.

ADAM: I'm not saying that you can't read this book and not—

MARGE: It's not more than that and maybe that's what I was getting. (11/24/2015)

Marge, in avoiding conflict with Adam, agrees that *The Cancer Journals* is "not more than" a "politically narrow feminist" view but also asks whether it is wrong to want to write a book with your own opinion. When I asked the group "Do you guys think anything that she says is sort of applicable to the HIV movement?" the conversation stopped. Diana responded, "Well that's an interesting question," and Adam added, "I didn't even ponder that." The group as a whole had a difficult time making connections between their work and memoirs that were not about HIV, even despite the key themes such as medical mistreatment and reckoning with death that Diana found so compelling. My question to the group is not unprecedented; Black gay writers like Joseph Beam and Essex Hemphill looked to Lorde's writing in the 1980s to find meaning in their own experience in the HIV crisis, a connection I have traced in previous work (Day 2007). What the group did discuss in relation to Audre Lorde's work and their own work with clients is the role of anger. Adam was adamant that Lorde was "mean" to hospital staff and connected this to his own experience as a practitioner.

DIANA: Well, maybe it was well deserved by that medical staff.

ADAM: Probably not. We see angry hurt people being very unkind to medical people on a regular basis.

NICK: Who they should be angry with is the drug companies and insurance companies.

MARGE: But they can't reach those people, that's why.

ADAM: Well what Diana was talking about we want a dichotomous world where there's good or bad, right or wrong, and it's too complex to boil it down to that. To get angry at this, to get angry at that. It's sad. It's tragic.

DIANA: Right, right.

ADAM: I'm sad for you. I don't know what causes it. Your genetics, what you ate in Grenada causes it; I don't know what causes it, it is just sad. And what are we going to do about it?

The group here uses xenophobic rhetoric ("what you ate in Grenada") to distance themselves from Lorde and to critique the overall utility of her anger. Their conversation about Lorde's anger leads them to make connections with their work experience within their ASO.

GRETTA: I was just thinking about a patient I had today that was very angry.
DIANA: Oh yah, talk about that.
GRETTA: They were angry because like they went to jail and was given medications incorrect medications.
DIANA: And he's only 28.
GRETTA: Yah, very very angry. They gave him one med and you need a cocktail whether or not that is in one med but you need a cocktail. And the doctor kept going back in and going back in and saying "I need meds" and so the doctor looked on his phone, googled, Truvada popped up and that is what he prescribed. And that does not work by itself.
DIANA: That doc is a civil liberties case, that's for damn sure.

The group here responds to Gretta with a sort of resigned familiarity with this kind of incompetence. Ultimately, the group agrees that the medical error is an unfair target of the affected patient.

GRETTA: Yeah. It's going to increase how the virus affects him and all this junk. But this makes me think of him—there is a point—because it is like fighting the system and he is pissed off at the jail, and he's mad at the doctor, and he's pissed off at us for not catching it earlier and yadayadayada but that's like, it is similar in the same way because he shouldn't be mad at the doctor he should be mad at the—I get that he has a case but he should be mad at society in general for not having any information, not having any medication about HIV and how medications work. Not that anybody can be a doctor but if we lived in a society where there wasn't so much stigma.

Gretta highlights a daily interaction with systemic injustice in relation to HIV and the prison system. This conversation reflects on stigma in relation to HIV and prison while reinforcing stigma by locating it in the individual responsibility of those with HIV to "just talk about it"— a prime example of how the political economy of stigma operates. Within the political economy of stigma, the individual is responsible for their own condition; by focusing on individual responsibility, systemic injustice is obscured. Gretta's discussion excuses an individual doctor's ignorance over systemic problems within the medical system:

GRETTA: It made me connect it to this [*The Cancer Journals*] because she was really angry at the system and I get that, he should be angry at the system too—no, he should be pissed off at that doctor, he should but he shouldn't because is it the doctor's fault that society has made it where doctors don't know that. Should he have done more research? Yah. But if we didn't hide everything medical then—I think I would be mad at the doctor too but at the same point, you know, by forcing him to become an advocate, the word survivor, is geared at breast cancer survivors then you have to be strong and powerful and pink and woohoo

DIANA: Exactly.

GRETTA: And I'm like, I feel like I do that to my patients a lot. I just want to shake them and be like "Why can't you just be out and open?" The statement about death, I say it to a lot of my patients, when they are talking about starting to come out and they tell people the first couple of people is really hard. Once you tell everyone, no one can do anything to you. Everyone knows. They are not going to because you are out!

NICK: Right, and that's my thing. Why do you want to surround yourself with people [who] are going to think negatively of you? I tell people, "weed out the bad."

GRETTA: Right. I, on the other hand, on the flip side, I am trying to force my patients to be advocates and I am trying to tell them "go out," you know, "say that you are positive!" Look at Marge, she goes into every single room and says that she is positive—

NICK: You are empowering your clients and that is how we will change the system.

What began with Diana challenging Adam that perhaps the medical team in charge of Lorde's care deserves Lorde's anger leads to a discussion of medical mismanagement disclosed by a client in prison and his anger. What is an interesting interpretation is that the group decides that the problem with the system of medical care is not the bureaucracy but ultimately the unwillingness of clients to disclose their HIV status. As Gretta says, once all her clients are out in the open, she will no longer need to be a clinical social worker. For this group, individual disclosure is the cure for a broken system. For Lorde in *The*

Cancer Journals, her individual disclosure is meant to reveal the brokenness but is not a cure in itself.

In the next chapter, I analyze the limits of disclosure within our current medical system in the US. Through the political economy of stigma, disclosure itself is produced and incorporated to reinforce stigma through diagnostic reading practices: not only can this practice limit the creativity of interpretive reading and medical practices; it can also be a form of exploitation through which the medical industrial complex can profit. Specifically, in the next chapter, I look at the growing practice of narrative medicine and its circulation of narrative as a medical commodity.[5]

---

5. I am using commodity here in much the same way Michelle Murphy does in *The Economization of Life*: "A commodity is more than just a thing for sale made of labor; it is also an object of desire, and even more, an object that has attached to it a larger surplus of circulating abstract desire that is in excess of the functionalist need for the specific object" (25).

CHAPTER 4

Privacy, Bioethics, and Narrative Medicine

Narrative disclosure has recently become the focus of medical practitioners, most significantly seen with the rise of programs in the medical humanities. As I mentioned in the introduction, I use this term *medical humanities,* which aims specifically to contribute a foundation of ethics, history, and the arts to formal medical education in order to impact physician practice (Shapiro et al.) to specifically contrast the term *health humanities,* which emerges to account for humanities scholars who think about the physiological experiences of health, disease, and disability within and beyond doctor–patient or other medicalized relationships, a field that Olivia Banner suggests can use disability studies itself as a central methodological tool (2019, 1–3). The medical humanities tends to focus on "instrumental imperatives" as opposed to "social, political, and cultural imperatives" in the health humanities (3). In previous chapters, I have compared reading groups of women living with HIV and ASO service workers, critiquing how each group reads and reacts to narrative given their relationships to medicine and diagnosis. Those chapters implicitly theorize the potential effect of these similar and often disparate reactions to narrative between patients and providers on the actual practice and effectiveness of medicine, ending with a reflection on the role of narrative in medical education. This chapter turns to the explicit adoption of narrative in medical education and questions its utility within the political economy of stigma.

In this chapter, I explore a prominent medical humanities program, Columbia University's Program in Narrative Medicine. I do so in order to analyze how deploying narrative expertise within neoliberal medical practices can harm individual patients and strengthen the very systems of oppression that programs in the medical humanities seek to destabilize. In setting a framework of the political economy of stigma in the previous chapters, explored through the reading practices and narratives of those living with HIV and of medical providers, we can already understand the stakes of deploying narrative—when it may be counterproductive and harmful for individuals, reinforcing systems of oppression for those with, to paraphrase Sontag, the most stigmatizing condition of our time.

Despite narrative's deployment within a social justice framework, we must still be cautious about fetishizing narrative within a profit-based medical model. In order to make this argument, I use the key practice of narrative medicine practitioners, close reading. I begin with Rita Charon's 2008 monograph *Narrative Medicine*. This book is often presented and read as a seminal text for the brand; *brand* is the term Charon herself uses in her introductions at the 2015 Narrative Medicine workshop I attended. I conduct this close reading in relation to theories of privacy and feminist critiques of the medical industrial complex in the US. Second, I explore my own experience attending a weekend-long Narrative Medicine workshop at Columbia University, geared toward practitioners as a continuing education credit. I do this in order to explore how narrative medicine becomes interpreted as both a pedagogical and a medical practice. Third, I theorize the circulation of writing about narrative medicine, including Charon's co-written 2017 monograph as well as other academic publications encouraging the adoption of narrative medicine at medical schools. Because this monograph is a book about books, in so many ways, I think it is methodologically congruent to closely read publications about narrative medicine *as* narrative itself, circulated within the same market systems.

Branding Close Reading, Problematizing Privacy

Through the political economy of stigma, we can understand that author–reader relationships are mediated by larger systemic industries, including the book publishing industry (explored in chapter 1) as well as for memoirs about disability and illness, the medical industry. As Tasha Dubriwny explains, under neoliberalism, medicine operates so that individual subjects are "free to construct their own lives" but do so within "prevailing market forces, and (in the United States) a healthcare system in which 40 million individuals are uninsured" (26). The Affordable Care Act addresses some issues of access to medical services, but not the underlying social inequalities that lead to long-term health concerns in economically and racially marginalized communities (164).[1] Even if someone who has been marginalized because of racism, classism, or sexism, as were many of the women living with HIV that I worked with, she may not have access to the narrative resources (education, literacy, cognitive normalcy) of more privileged patients and of doctors themselves, reinforcing an unbalanced power dynamic often critiqued by women's health activists in the 1970s and 1980s. As Dubriwny theorizes, medical subjects are offered two things within neoliberalism: consumption and surveillance (153). Narrative medicine directly plays into this consumption (doctors, reading public) and surveillance (patients, writing public), reinforcing neoliberal subjectivity within the medical industrial complex.

Background about how the medical industrial complex constructs subjectivity within neoliberalism is important for understanding the recent rise of the medical humanities, and in one particular brand of the medical humanities, narrative medicine. Rita Charon, creator and medical practitioner, defines narrative medicine not as a specialty within medical practice but as "medicine practiced with the narrative competence to recognize, absorb, interpret, and be moved by the stories of illness" (ii).[2] It is not a coincidence that Charon begins to theorize the importance of first-person accounts of illness at a time when these are flying off bookstore shelves during the memoir boom. One of the goals of narrative medicine, as elaborated in her 2008 monograph, is to provide tools for doctors to be more humane and ethical in the practice of medicine (ii). It is a clinical practice "informed by the theory and practice of reading, writing, telling and receiving stories" (ii–iii). For Charon, this is about countering the practice of "eight-minute visits" and insurance's bottom line. While wanting to extend the time that patients spend with doctors face to face is on the surface admirable, and something health humanities scholar Delese Wear has been advocating in the form of "slow medicine," the problem of insurance companies using time as part of an algorithm for charging more for those visits means that the practice of longer visits and use of patient narrative will occur only for those affluent enough to afford it, further alienating and disenfranchising those who are poor (Wear and Zarconi).[3] A key problem with narrative medicine is that it addresses what has fallen out of practice in

---

1. In the conclusion, I look more closely at recent funding cuts to the Ryan White Program and how this directly affects who gets care and what care means.

2. Charon holds both an MD in internal medicine and a PhD in English literature.

3. For more on the structure of insurance company pricing, please read Elizabeth Rosenthal, *An American Sickness: How Healthcare Became Big Business and How You Can Take It Back* (Penguin, 2017).

medicine (one-on-one relationships with doctors built over time) but not who has fallen out of medical care. Narrative medicine does nothing to address the larger structural issues of medical practice that is based on a profit model. What it does do is draw narrative expertise into the medical industrial complex and reinforce the existing power dynamics where medical practitioners also become narrative experts. This is not because of the intention of the practitioner but because the problems of the deeply unequal system of medical practice in the US have not been disrupted.

As Charon writes, promoting her own Ivy League courses in narrative medicine, "although everyone grows up listening to and telling stories, sophisticated knowledge of how stories work is not attained without considerable effort and commitment" (ix). While Charon does elaborate on a taxonomy of five narrative components for clinicians to analyze in their close reading of patient stories—frame, form, time, plot, desire (114–27)—she continually refers to the goal of recognizing a "universality" of the "human condition." She writes explicitly, "Let us revel in the inexhaustibility of our combinations and the universality of our relations, our affiliations, our common burdens, and gifts as we do our best to heal" (xiii); thus, while Charon emphasizes the complexity of narrative and the need for medical expertise in evaluating patient narrative, her goals remain problematic. As I have argued in previous work, postcolonial feminist theory is useful for interpretation here (Day 2011). In her essay on reading the archives for historical information about colonized subjects, Gayatri Spivak maintains that what we don't know is as much a part of the story as what we do (1985, 247–72). Spivak's key argument is that we should read the archives not as a simplistic representation of a linear narrative story but as an interrupted narrative much more about the creator of the archive than about the purported subject (251). Spivak argues that it is exactly these gaps, these incongruences, in the historical record that can provide us an understanding of the colonized subject (268–71). I argue that to truly transform power relationships in medicine, we need to value what we don't know. Instead of asking for more information from marginalized clients, we should value the gaps in disclosure and be attentive to our own assumptions about how entitled we are to client narrative detail. While I agree with many of the critiques of health humanities scholars Rebecca Garden, Delese Wear, and Olivia Banner in their calls for reading for open-endedness, my argument is slightly different. I propose that the valorization of narrative itself is problematic because of what I am calling the *narrative entitlement* of doctors (and others in positions of power and privilege); narrative entitlement is a term I created to connote the relationship in which a medical provider feels that they are owed narrative details of a client-patient's life, regardless of whether those details impact treatment options. Narrative entitlement is an effect of a larger system of inequality that has conceived of individual privacy as a privilege. Narrative entitlement is an effect of White patriarchal cisgender, able-bodied privilege that is now capitalized on within a neoliberal medical market. Narrative medicine is a beneficiary of this privilege.

As Karla Holloway reminds us, privacy is a privilege that "legal and medical interest in identity obscures. [. . .] Liberty cannot be a claim to individuality when individual identity is filtered through our associations and assignments to identity categories" (2011, 20). Yet narrative medicine focuses on the individual body, and while being attentive to "cultural difference" and poverty might help a clinician be a good person and make a swifter medical diagnosis, the limitations of the parameters of medicine, and of the medical industrial complex, cannot be solved.

In her book-length interrogation of private personhood and bioethics, Holloway inadvertently makes an argument against narrative medicine when she writes of her methodology: "Unlike law and medicine, fiction is free to indulge its complications rather than constrained to rigorous enforcement of boundaries that encourage expeditious resolution" (10). Not only is medicine limited by its focus on resolution (or diagnosis, containment, cure), which often relies on understanding identity as fixed and diagnostic, as opposed to differential, mobile, and ambiguous, but it also contributes to the valorization and circulation of narrative as a product for profit, negating privacy and upholding the political economy of stigma.

Reading Foucault's lectures at College de France, Holloway synthesizes that in sovereignty, the subject is never an individualized body (xvi). Holloway contends that "the objectification of a patient's story fails to give a constitutive weight to the cultural and historical context of that experience" (xvii). Thus, Holloway focuses her analysis on how identities interact in the public sphere, not individuals (7). Holloway's reading resists the individualism that Charon's practice relies on, providing a useful analysis on the limits of narrative medicine. For Holloway, narrative medicine cannot "ignore the intersections of science, medicine, law and society" (xvii). It is precisely within the political economy of stigma that narrative medicine emerges, individualizing medical experience as distinct from—though, importantly, affected by—systems of intersectional oppression. I argue that the latter is important in narrative medicine pedagogy because forms of oppression become valuable signifiers to be collected by the practitioner in the form of a narrative commodity but not something that influences the practitioners to change the diagnostic structures of medical care itself. The medical subject is still a patient who is subject to and interpreted through a memoir industry unpacked in my first chapter. The doctor, through narrative medicine practice, can demonstrate their social justice commitment through branding. This branding happens by demonstrating previous success in collecting stories of the oppressed.

Whereas Holloway writes about privacy as a privilege not afforded to those marginalized by gender and class, Carrie Griffin Basas applies understandings of privacy directly to disability identity, reminding us that "the law is not the same for everyone, especially when viewed through the lenses of disability [. . .]. When their privacy needs are espoused, they are to mask abuses and injustices committed against them by the state or private actors" (187). In arguing that privacy laws have been used to protect the interests of the state and other able-bodied actors, Basas highlights how disabled people as a group have been made "voiceless" (189). In analyzing how the Americans with Disability Act has operated in the last twenty-five years, Basas finds that private issues for people with disabilities become public for "fact finders, judges and jurors" (191). It is not simply in cases of ADA litigation that people with disabilities relinquish privacy; they routinely do so to access the US public benefits program (192): "If a person wants financial support from the government, he or she must be willing to relinquish some privacy—money is traded for probing" (192). The contradiction here is that people with disabilities are consistently having their privacy expunged for the sake of proving disability to access public resources; yet, when people with disabilities accuse businesses and other private actors of discrimination or abuse, those private actors are protected by their privacy (187–93). What is important here is that narrative medicine emerges precisely through these dynamics, where "money is traded for probing" for the sake of enhancing an already biased (in some cases, abusive) medical system.

Working within the field of cultural ethics, Holloway excavates patterns produced in narratives; one important pattern is the conceptualization and value of what is considered "private," as the private relates to race, age, ability, and gender. As such, the private is used as a lens through which to interrogate identity, bioethics, and narrative (xvii–xx). Ultimately, as Holloway contends, privacy is a "socially selective privilege" (2011, 7). As Holloway writes, "Privacy has a value that is intimately attached to the history of our laws, as well as to the social evolution of our attitudes regarding difference. Gender and race have particular (arguably, peculiar) legal histories in the United States that make the idea of privacy read differently for different bodies. [. . .] Social values and social systems are critical dimensions of science and medicine" (6). The socially selective privilege is not something afforded to people with chronic illness and disability, as Basas argues. Narrative medicine is another means through which privacy is negated.

What is useful about narrative medicine is that it teaches clinicians to "tolerate ambiguity and identify the unspoken subtexts" (Charon 4); Charon's work is in direct conversation with the theories of pain that Elaine Scarry and others have developed: pain and suffering can be impossible to actually put into words or narrative (4). At the same time that Charon recognizes the value of ambiguity, she contradicts this value: to "know what patients endure at the hands of illness and therefore to be of clinical help requires that doctors enter the world of their patients, if only imaginatively, and to see and interpret these worlds from their patients' point of view" with the goal of "illuminating the universals of the human condition" (9). In other words, clinicians must be able to identify with patients and put themselves in their place instead of what postcolonial feminist theorists might ask, which is to value the inability to know. "Using narrative competence, caretakers can do what anyone who witnesses suffering does—in a family, among friends, in the news, on the stage, in fiction, on the street, in the hospital—one knows, one feels, one responds, and one *joins with* the one who suffers" (12). Here, Charon relies on a simplistic understanding of witnessing, an understanding that is often critiqued. As cultural theorist Lauren Berlant argues, witnessing and compassion imply a relationship between the spectator and sufferer where the emphasis is on the spectator's feeling (2004, 1). Compassion itself is a social and aesthetic technology of belonging, not an "organic emotion" (5). In medicine, this reinforces the top-down power dynamic. As Berlant argues, when compassion is understood as an emotion, the scale of the ethical response is individualized (6). Psychiatrist and scholar Jonathan Metzl similarly cautions us against this kind of individualizing of structural problems within medicine, arguing that even programs intended to address "cultural competency" within medicine tend to exacerbate uneven power dynamics by misrepresenting and oversimplifying culture, conflating culture with race (and reinforcing racism) and leaving medical culture largely without scrutiny (200–201). Metzl writes, "Racialized assumptions and biases are historically embedded into the very DNA of healthcare delivery systems and shape interactions and outcomes largely before participants appear on the scene. As such, I believe that focusing on the individual obscures the impact of the structural, while putting undue pressure on even well-intentioned patients or doctors to solve problems in ten-minute office visits that have taken decades or even centuries to evolve" (202). Narrative medicine contributes to this neoliberal individualization of health and illness with a focus on diagnosis, not social justice, reinforcing the political economy of stigma.

Olivia Banner recently critiques narrative medicine within the larger project of the medical humanities, writing that the interpretive processes of the medical humanities are part of the problem. Citing the work of Brian Dolan, Banner looks at how the medical humanities emerges after the Reagan administration slashes National Endowment for the Humanities funding in 1981; the medical humanities was a field justified to add value to medical education at a time when the humanities in general was devalued and underfunded (2017, 15). Banner writes: "It is against this history that I view key medical humanities principles such as developing empathy and listening. The goals of improving individuals' interpersonal skills are often enlisted to address issues that to my mind are caused by deep structural problems—a typical neoliberal technique to depoliticize what are social and economic issues" (13). Banner argues that medical schools use medical humanities as way to counter critiques of health care more generally and that empathy becomes something quantified within the logic of the market itself; later in this chapter I look at precisely this phenomenon in the circulation of narrative medicine practice abroad.

By incorporating acts of witnessing and compassion into medicine, Charon adds another limitation to these acts by incorporating it into systems of diagnosis: "The diagnostic act requires two contradictory impulses at once: the effort to register the unique features of that which is observed and the simultaneous act to categorize it to make it 'readable'" (46). In order to conduct this twofold act, Charon encourages practitioners to keep a "parallel chart" where they journal about patients because "if they can capture it with greater force and accuracy, it means they are perceiving it more accurately and more fully as it occurs. The writing not only helps them answer the call of patient suffering but helps them hear it. This is very radical" (139). At the same time that Charon writes of this parallel chart-keeping as radical (alluding that this changes the power dynamics in medicine), she also emphasizes the need for doctors to "call forth the authentic in one another" (33–35), without any sort of explanation of what *authentic* means. In Charon's explication of narrative medicine, there is nothing that changes the power dynamics of doctor–patient relationships—what emerges through keeping a parallel chart is the focus on making doctors more efficient practitioners (avoiding mistakes in diagnosis and treatment by listening more carefully, increasing their own powers of observation, particularly when there are differences in cultural practices and language) as opposed to inviting patients into the diagnostic process and actually shifting the power dynamics in medicine.

In her final discussion of narrative medicine, which is focused on bioethics, Charon discusses how narrative reframes bioethics because it requires bioethics to be understood as "an enterprise in which one subject enters relation with another subject, both participants in the inter-subjectivity illuminating one another's goals, hopes, desires, and fears, and contributing regard, trust and courage" (208). Yet none of the techniques Charon explicates reflect intersubjectivity. This can be attributed to the broader limitations of practicing medicine within the medical industrial complex.

We must understand narrative medicine as a circulated product within the medical industrial complex and as an effect of the political economy of stigma and the very privilege it seeks to destabilize. Like all effects of privilege, narrative medicine is part of a systemic problem, regardless of the intention of practitioners. Banner writes that the medical humanities has a complete absence of understandings of race; narrative medicine itself operates under the hypothesis that practices used to "foster empathy" will improve medical practice when, in fact, these practices are more apt to exacerbate medical racism (21–25). In what follows, I show precisely how this happens through the pedagogy of narrative medicine. As long as medicine is still conducted using a for-profit model, where patient well-being is always subordinated to a cost-benefit analysis, then narrative can never function ethically—it merely erodes privacy, particularly from the most marginalized bodies.

Narrative Medicine—From Close Reading to Pedagogy

My close reading of Rita Charon's foundational 2008 book, *Narrative Medicine*, raised several questions that stem from my feminist disability studies background. In an initial review of my writing about Charon's book, a mentor challenged me, saying, "These are good people, aren't they?" She pushed me to do more exploration in this practice that is attempting to address social injustice. This mentor was referring to practitioners of narrative medicine, highlighting distinctions between my institutional critiques and the well-meaning individuals who are seeking ethical foundations for their own medical practice. I took this mentor's observation to heart and began to construct a field research study. Over the course of the following year, amid my first full-time teaching job and field research with AIDS service workers, I wrote a grant and procured the funds to attend a weekend-long Narrative Medicine Workshop at Columbia University Medical School (the workshop fees alone were $850, a cost far beyond my capacity as a first-year public university professor). From the outset, I was excited about the conference; I had interviewed the Narrative Medicine program director and found him friendly and open to my attendance as a disability studies scholar (an unfamiliar field to him). I was still skeptical, but my anger had vanished; I was looking for places of coalition between narrative medicine and disability studies.

A month before my departure, I was attending another academic conference, where I met a graduate student enrolled in Columbia's Public Health program. When I mentioned that I would be in her neck of the woods for a narrative medicine workshop, she responded, "Oh I loooooooooove narrative medicine! You know, I didn't think of it in relation to disabled people, but I am sure it would be so therapeutic for them!" I took a bite of my vegetable dumpling, smiled, and changed the topic. The problem with this student's response was the automatic assumption that people with disabilities are looking for therapy and have nothing to offer in intellectual service to narrative medicine practitioners. While I had slowly shrugged off my self-righteous assumptions about narrative medicine over the course of the year, this interaction put me on guard again, warning me that I would have work to do in explaining disability studies as a field and my critiques of some of the epistemological assumptions of narrative medicine.

During the conference I kept a participant observation journal, a practice encouraged among all conference attendees. In what follows, I summarize some of the material from that journal, highlighting important pedagogical strategies of the workshop and participant and facilitator reactions to my own participation. Before the workshop, participants were sent a schedule and PDFs of two readings: the first was a 2011 essay by Shannon Wooden on teaching *The Curious Incident of the Dog in the Night-Time* through a narrative medicine and disability studies lens (the second reading, which I describe later, was a short story by Salinger). I did my best to set my cynicism aside and dive right in.

I was terribly disappointed.

Wooden begins by discussing narrative ethics and how narrative medicine can be used as a tool to teach ethical reading. In introducing the project, she highlights the importance to disability studies but fails to use anything from disability studies to think through the ethics of reading practices. Wooden "invites" her undergraduate students to read Mark Haddon's novel like a medical doctor because "this puts us in a position where we must practice empathy" and avoid ethical judgments. I can't help but think about the many ways in which reading as a practitioner invites ethical judgment because implicitly the practitioner is called to intervene in some way. And then Wooden encourages her students to read with a diagnosis in mind, reminding us that this is, of course, not a medical narrative. Additionally, she characterizes Christopher, the main character, several times as a child "with special needs" who has an "inability to understand" what is going on in the text around him (279). The latter is not a new literary phenomenon—in high school we talked at length about *The Great Gatsby*'s Nick and his unreliable narration, a naïveté that makes him unable to understand some of what is happening in the text— but what makes it irritating in this article is that the inability is connected to autism, to disability itself. It is assumed that it is the autism that obscures understanding as opposed to the social conditions that shape the textual world of the narrator. Neurodivergency does not de facto lead to "misunderstanding" or naïveté, though many autism self-advocates have commented on this form of common sense enacted in relationships with medical professionals.[4]

Wooden spends much of the essay discussing the role of Christopher's parents, whom readers come to sympathize with because, as she writes, "it becomes very difficult to imagine taking care of a child with such difficult circumstances as his disability presents" (280). In fact, Wooden asks students to avoid "political correctness" (and she conflates identity politics with political correctness, missing that feminist and critical race theorists are identifying multiple and intersecting systems of oppression) and identify suffering in the book—and, indeed, suffering is understood as individual here, related to the condition of autism, and not political, related to structural ableism (or even medicine itself) (282). About halfway through the essay, the author brings in a disability studies theorist, Michael Bérubé. Unfortunately, she quotes Bérubé out of context, writing, "most of our culture is socially constructed along the medical model to begin with" in order to argue that it doesn't take much for a teacher of *The Curious Incident* to use it as a medical text (282–83). Bérubé's writing that our culture is constructed along a medical model is a critique of diagnostic practices, not a promotion of them. While quoting Bérubé later in his text, Wooden misses a key analysis he provides in his introduction, where he asks readers explicitly not to diagnose characters, "reading with the DSM-V" (20), explicating that disability studies is not concerned in literature with the individual diagnosis of characters. Despite this framework that Bérubé provides for his own work, Wooden says that by reading *The Curious Incident* diagnostically, "we become attuned to the text's many salient concrete details—even the unpleasant and deliberately minimized ones" (283). She encourages students to read with a DSM-IV-TR handy (283). She references one critique of a neuroqueer person reflecting that *The Curious Incident* is not representative of his/her own experience but fails to highlight the larger neuroqueer community out of which this critique comes and is widely reflective (285).

And then another confusing thing happens. Wooden asks students to "define the spectrum broadly"—in essence falling into a trap of "we are all disabled sometimes"—and continues to misplace the political implications of structural oppression that the novel does highlight. She goes on to reference Couser and Frank, encouraging students to read beyond diagnosis and to recognize that this story is a "triumphant narrative" (287)—failing to draw on any

---

4. See, for instance, Yergeau; Nicolaidis; Johnson.

disability studies scholarship that critiques our understandings of triumph. In fact, in her ableist reading of *The Curious Incident,* she says that reading triumphantly will counterbalance what "most of her students feel" at the end of the novel, who "report feeling despair" because "readers remain skeptical of his [Christopher's] college plans, too, or any notion of his being independent, self-sufficient, or happy" (288).

To be fair, Wooden begins to locate ableism and the social constructions of disability toward the end of her critique, somewhat haphazardly, and then asserts that a narrative medicine reading forces us to confront our own ableism—and I have yet to figure out how this works, based on her own arguments. Finally, though, I was relieved to see her assert that while we can use categories for diagnosis in our reading, we should also be critiquing those categories (maybe she could begin her article with this statement and then start over entirely?). All of these initial thoughts regarding our first reading leave me 80 percent frustrated and 20 percent curious about the reaction and small group discussions in relation to disability studies.

The second item we were asked to read in advance was Salinger's short story "For Esmé—with Love and Squalor"; in my overview of syllabi from the Narrative Medicine program, I find that this is a typical selection for class close readings: a short story by a White male with whom American readers may already be familiar. In a practice about collecting life stories, Narrative Medicine primarily assigns fiction. I believe in my own classrooms that pedagogy begins with the curation of course materials: that what materials are included and in what order essentially tells students who belongs in the class and why. From the beginning of my experience in the workshop, I understood that a neurodivergent person would be unwelcome from the first reading; from the second reading, I understood that someone without a White American middle-class background would easily be left behind if they were unfamiliar with Salinger and suspected that if someone had [feminist crip] critiques of Salinger, they, too, might feel misplaced.

During the opening plenary, Rita Charon introduces the workshop, tells us that it has evolved over the years because "we know more now and you know more" but also that the brand is the same; she reiterates that narrative medicine is a "brand" of the medical humanities. Here, I look around, hoping to make eye contact with someone who will recognize this allegiance to the neoliberal university—we no longer have fields of study, we have brands. Everyone is facing diligently forward. No eye contact is made.

We spend time together looking at three Rothko paintings (the assumption is that everyone is sighted) and she talks about our "capacities for attention"; she talks about how we have to "donate one's presence"—which I think is an ironic use of the word *donate* since we all paid to be here. She asks us to pay attention to the "thing" the story "does" (I like this idea). She ends by asking the group what it would take to turn the health-care system around. She says she is not a political organizer but that we need to combat the pharma industry and the insurance industry, and, in many ways, I am hooked. The problem is that Charon never tells us how narrative medicine will undo these industries; in the process, she seems to create a bifurcation between political organization and a capacity to care for patients.

The second day includes smaller breakout sessions where racism and sexism become apparent. For example, we are asked to write about our names. One woman describes the debates between her Guatemalan father and Jewish mother in the 1970s. An older White psychiatrist in the group responds, "I thought you were Indian, so pretty," and neither the facilitator nor any group participants call this psychiatrist out for his remarks. What I understand here as a sexist and Orientalizing subjectivity is accepted as an interpersonal norm for the group; those who notice it are uneasy about unsettling the group dynamics, being a feminist killjoy, while others undoubtedly are so used to such comments that they don't notice it. As an educator of social justice, I would be remiss not to address a comment like this in my own classroom. I understand now that in this workshop, there are different standards.

Ableism within the workshop was also immediately apparent: people with disabilities were objects of laughter or curiosity. For example, in these same small breakout groups, we read a 2010 Nellie Herman short story which begins with a "joke" about confusing a baby with a midget on a billboard. Everyone is laughing. I am not quite understanding the joke, but I pretend to laugh too. I want to seem part of the club. After reading the first half we are asked to each spend a few minutes writing what we believe is the end of the story. I remember doing exercises like this in my intro creative writing courses in college. We share our alternative endings with one another. When our workshop leader asks us to reflect on the exercise, the group members all say that it was fun and that so far, the weekend has been fun because they all came here to work on their writing skills. I am in a group of eight others, all physicians or psychiatrists, one filmmaker. In sharing with my partner, a pediatric physician about my age, that I am a disability studies professor, she responds, "Oh I read your bio! You must get a lot of interesting stories to write about," and I am wondering what it is she thinks I do.

We never address the critical article about *Curious Incident*; there is no content that would address strategies for bridging cultural differences, language barriers, or disabled bodies. We spend the day practicing our own creative writing.

The next morning, we work in small groups on listening skills—we are meant to tell a "traumatic" story from our lives [I tell the story of my geriatric deaf-blind dog escaping in the month following a move; my partner tells the story of needing to fire her nanny] and reflect on what it feels like to be listened to. When we come back together to report, and two groups talk about the stories where people with disabilities are centered—the "trauma" is that the storyteller is the "caregiver." When we are all giving feedback, I go last and try to avoid talking; I am overwhelmed with the ableism in the telling, the assumption of the tellers that the people with disability in their stories do not have their own perspectives, and that the very act of living with someone, providing care for someone with a disability, is a traumatic experience. Finally, I confess my hesitations. I use the word *ableist.* The group asks me for a definition. I am asked whether that is even a real word. There is skepticism in the room. Later, the group leader, an English professor and member of the NM faculty, singles me out in front of the group, telling me that I am being too critical, that perhaps the program is not concerned enough with social justice for me but for everyone else, it is working just fine. I am, in Sara Ahmed's formulation, the feminist killjoy.[5] Later, I will email this professor, thanking her for her comments, asking whether she wouldn't mind answering a few questions about her involvement with NM as a field; she responds immediately and what I read as enthusiastically. I send the questions. I never hear back.

The weekend workshop ends with a plenary on narrative ethics. The speaker lectures on his use of photography and speaks for nearly forty-five minutes with the picture of a disabled woman of color climbing the stairs displayed behind him. He speaks about how he asked his patients, this woman being one of them, if he could photograph them not in his capacity as a doctor but as a citizen. This woman evidently agreed, though I wonder if she understood that her photograph would be used in a medical school workshop. He speaks about how "witnessing" people in their homes opened up his empathy as a doctor; I am wondering why he isn't angry that this disabled woman of color is forced because of income to live in an inaccessible apartment building. He says he now understands why she doesn't leave her house as often, why she doesn't exercise. I don't believe you need to follow a patient home to gain that

---

5. Sara Ahmed has written about how this figure of the feminist killjoy is the feminist who is seen, in naming the problem, as the cause of the problem; in noticing, you are doing political work but in naming what you notice, you become the problem and are often discredited through being labeled as too emotional (31–42). Ahmed writes, "When you are alienated by virtue of how you are affected, you are an affect alien. A feminist killjoy is an affect alien. We are not made happy by the right things" (57).

understanding; I certainly don't think you need to have her photo displayed, faceless, for a room full of practitioners.

What does it mean that narrative medicine is conceptualized as a "brand"? What does it mean that my questions about ableism are considered inconvenient? That the existence of the term *ableism* in itself is questioned? That in all the attention the workshop paid to close reading, we only ever read "well-told" stories—in fact, as one workshop leader and NM faculty member told us, it is only through well-told stories that we can learn close reading. Why did we not read and practice close listening with people with disabilities or illness? What does it mean that in a closing plenary we can sit in front of a picture of a nameless, faceless disabled woman of color for forty-five minutes in a discussion about ethics and no one questions the ethics of that photograph? No one visibly squirms in their seat?

About six months later, I pose these questions at another interdisciplinary conference with disability studies scholars and medical humanities scholars in conjunction with some initial findings from my AIDS service workers field research. The person chairing my panel is a psychiatrist from an elite university. She is visibly angry with me, speaking in short quick clips and a carefully modulated voice. She says after the panel that Columbia's Narrative Medicine program is doing good work, that she is hosting a lunchtime talk about gentrification in her university's neighborhood. That I simply do not understand but that of course, we need to be more inclusive of disabled people. I am nodding as she speaks, attempting to keep a calm façade through our brief interaction, though I am visibly frustrated—perhaps with her interpretations of my work, perhaps with my own inability to communicate and persuade those invested in narrative medicine of their participation in the political economy of stigma.

A fellow colleague approaches me after the panel, tells me how relieved she is that I finally verbalized what she has been struggling to articulate: this idea that the problem with the medical humanities as a whole is the focus on the stories of those with privilege, asking doctors and medical students to participate in self-reflection without actually asking clients, patients, those in multiply marginalized positions for their perspective. I am relieved that my talk worked—that this audience member understood that the problem is not going to be solved by simply adding a few disabled people to a stew and stirring; the recipe needed to be changed entirely.

My analysis here of participating in a narrative medicine workshop is admittedly anecdotal, falling in line with much of Charon's own writing in her 2008 monograph; it is participant observation, and likely other disability studies scholars or feminist studies scholars could participate and find different results. Yet, my critique resonates with others. Filmmaker and English literature scholar Emily Reach, in a 2013 TED Talk, makes a similar observation about the limitations of narrative medicine. In her reading and at NM conferences, Reach observes,

> I began to notice that when people talk about narrative they really mean only one of two things: they are talking about narrative as a diagnostic tool—so like think of the show *House* here—narrative is something that doctors can use so that if they can understand their patient's life stories better, they can get to a diagnosis more quickly; or they are talking about this idea of narrative as a therapeutic tool, so that stories are things that patients tell themselves in order to cope with their diseases, especially when they know they are not going to get better.

Similar to Reach, in my experience with narrative medicine, I was both an outsider as a nonphysician (though there were a few other humanities folks in the group of sixty participants) and an insider as a White, well-educated, apparently able-bodied, cisgender woman. What concerns me with my experience in this narrative medicine workshop is the lack of critical cultural analysis within which stories emerge; the lack of critical cultural theory that has developed around and through (life) narrative; and the continued practice of "branding" as listening to patients' stories as both a means to create medical expertise and a means through which medical practitioners can become published writers.

Medical practitioners are encouraged in these workshops to work on their writing skills above all other skills, and this expectation is reflected in the satisfaction of the participants. Narrative medicine practitioners can work on refining their writing for the process of publishing their patient stories through the auspices of narrative medicine.[6] I return again to Couser and his consideration of medical ethics and life writing, cited first in my introduction. Couser emphasizes the relationship between subject and reader, acknowledging that the more vulnerable the subject of life writing, the higher the ethical stakes (14–33). Couser argues that life writing should be an exercise of privacy, not a negation of it, meaning that the subject (whether someone is writing about their own experience of the experience of someone else) should be able to maintain some control of the material, maintaining private information (18–19). The call for medical practitioners to get as much detail as possible from their clients and then to craft their writing around that material, even while keeping patients anonymous, is a direct violation of this ethical

---

6. See, for example, DasGupta and Hurst.

principle. Further, Couser proposes the need for transparency between writer and subject—that a subject should know they are being written about. "The agreement of a subject to confide in a collaborator or life writer, then, is not carte blanche, not a waiver of privacy rights, but rather a willing sacrifice of privacy with the goal and expectation of some compensatory benefit" (22–23). Do narrative medicine practitioners disclose to their patients that they may write about them someday? That they want to be writers? That they want to publish? Respect for a subject of life writing includes understanding the subject themselves as a "source of literary property with potential market value" (24). Can one simultaneously treat a patient while thinking about the market value of their story? Part of the ethics of life writing that Couser calls for is transactional visibility, to make clear to readers how any story was obtained and circulated (25). If the first tenet of life-writing ethics is about transparency between writer and subject, the second tenet is about transparency between writer and reader. The political economy of stigma intentionally obscures a transparent relationship between reader and author as well as author and subject. Finally, according to Couser, an ethics of life writing must be accountable to a community, causing no harm or only justifiable harm—in other words, if one experiences discomfort or pain through life writing, that discomfort or pain must prove to be commensurate with the amount of good that life writing can do (30). Is the collection of narrative within the practice of narrative medicine able to be ethical? And can this translate within a neoliberal branding structure?

The Branding and Expansion of Narrative Medicine

In 2017 the faculty of the Program in Narrative Medicine at Columbia University co-wrote a pedagogical monograph, *The Principles and Practices of Narrative Medicine*. The book weaves together theoretical ideas expanded from Charon's original 2008 book alongside practical applications for teaching narrative medicine, compiling examples from their own workshop and classroom experience, primarily at Columbia but also in some international contexts. I read this new monograph after already writing the main ideas from this chapter and, admittedly, found myself holding my breath as I read to find what of my original critique might still hold.

Each chapter of the collection is written by one or two faculty members who contribute their insights from various fields of expertise; for example, Craig Irvine writes about Cartesian dualism in the medical field from his perspective as a continental philosopher, Maura Spiegel writes about literature from her perspective as an English PhD. As one might expect, my reading of this monograph was a mixed experience. In part III, I look more closely at the pieces of the monograph that allowed me to breathe, gave me space to think differentially about applications of narrative medicine. Here, I want to focus on a few tenets of my critique thus far that are amplified in this 2017 praxis.

The first amplification is the overall emphasis on the value of the literary. Maura Spiegel and Danielle Spencer begin the monograph with the chapter "Accounts of the Self: Exploring Relationality through Literature" (15–36). They begin by citing a recent study that finds those who read fiction perform better "on tests measuring theory of mind, social perception, and emotional intelligence after reading literary fiction. Notably, those who read nonfiction or popular fiction did not perform as well" (16). This study, with its raced, classed, gendered, and ableist implications for particular kinds of readings (who reads "literary fiction" and who determines what is literary? How are people of color, immigrants, non-native English speakers, people with disability left out of this population, and why?) and particular kinds of brains (what is "correct" social perception and who determines that? What is "emotional intelligence" and how is that determined by sanist ablest standards of performance?) becomes the basis for arguing why literary fiction is important for medical practitioners. Spiegel and Spencer go on to write about the importance of not reading books about medical care or illness precisely because doing so would be distracting, too invitational to a diagnostic reading, perhaps (16–18). There is also the explicit assumption that medical interaction mirrors all human interaction; the two write, "Much of healthcare happens in the interpersonal moments, and narrative medicine is attentive to the relational dynamics at work in every human encounter. In the medical context—and in any context—there is no such thing as a neutral human presence. [. . .] In the examination room, as in any room, an atmosphere is created between two people" (18). Posing the assumption that medical interaction is just like other human interaction presupposes that clients approach their doctors as they would a friend—no waiting room, no insurance infrastructure managing the clock, no white coat. Working on this assumption elides the differences that make medical interactions complex, exploitative, and expensive. Moreover, Spiegel and Spencer write about silence of a client as exhibiting a "need to tell" (20), exhibiting precisely the entitlement to narrative that I critiqued above. All of this is framed within the idea that literary fiction makes one better able to be attentive to and receive stories. My own research would show a precise opposite dynamic, particularly when understood through the creative economy of stigma that mediates reader-audience relations within the medical model.

Within *The Principles and Practice of Narrative Medicine,* Charon writes the chapter "Close Reading: The Signature Method of Narrative Medicine" (157–79). Already, by referring to the idea of a field having a "signature" method, Charon is ascribing a model of branding to her theoretical approach, critiqued above. Charon begins the chapter by emphasizing why we need close reading. She writes, "Despite the range of sources and skills bent toward the effort to improve clinical listening, patients continue to complain that their doctors, at least, don't listen to them, and so patients find their way to alternative healers, even if they need to pay directly for their services, *because* these practitioners are better able to attend to what they say" (158). Here, Charon presents an understanding that the reason patients would leave medical care is that a doctor lacks listening skills, not because of the structure of medicine itself as mandated by insurance structures, pharmaceutical companies, and other profit models. There is also the explicit assumption that alternative medical practitioners (acupuncturists, naturopaths, etc.) do not have an effective set of practices but simply are better listeners. The latter assumption carries with it a history of East versus West orientalism that devalues thousand-year-old practices and reduces practitioner expertise.[7] This assumption is also embedded in the very use of language like *alternative* or *complementary* medicine. With this framework, Charon traces the history of the rise of close reading in literature and then demonstrates how it reinforces the principles of narrative medicine (Action Toward Social Justice, Disciplinary Rigor, Inclusivity, Tolerating Ambiguity, Participatory and Non-hierarchical Methods, and Relational and Inter-subjective Processes) (171–75). Charon argues that close reading allows one to be attentive to one's own processes of meaning-making (170), a practice that closely mirrors the racist and ableist principles that stories of others are meant to make us know more about ourselves.

In applying close reading practices to health-care practice, Charon writes of an experience treating a client with a new diabetes diagnosis (271–85). She shares with readers excerpts from her notes about this client that she wrote and mailed to her. She begins, "Two middle-aged women sit in a cramped clinic office in upper Manhattan. They have known one another for decades, one of them moving through a series of health reversals and accomplishments and the other, as her doctor, accompanying her through them" (271). She moves on to describe the two women in all their similarities, having been Vietnam War activists and "taken to the streets with Our Bodies Ourselves" (272). Of the new diabetes diagnosis, Charon writes of her client's anxiety and distress; she writes about her client's self-discipline at having been active,

---

7. For more about this, see Harrington.

eaten well. "Perhaps, the doctor ventures, the elevated sugar was caused by this bad viral infection. That happens regularly." The emphasis here is on the possibility of a wrong or impermanent diagnosis—there is no recognition of the ableist, classed, and raced dynamics of a diabetes diagnosis itself, merely that this client should not be part of that picture (272–73). Instead, both seem to agree, in Charon's account, that diabetes signifies mortality:

> Even working in a hospital, as I do, I do not daily, actively confront the limits of my own life. But through the agency of my patient's merciless honesty about her mortality, I too underwent a graphic face-off with my not-too-far-off death [. . .] By accepting, consciously, that I share with patients the status of living-toward-death, we, together, somehow, see in the inevitability of a death to come the wordless worth of the life to come. (274)

Charon gives one example to emphasize that doctors can and should show clients their meeting notes and look for moments where they can find similarities with their patients.

> So, as we sat together at my desk we looked at one another with recognition, a reciprocal recognition in which we become mirrors for one another at the same time that we are both doctor and patient. The fact that we shared some actual features of life as politically active women professors in our sixties living in Manhattan may have quickened the process of reciprocal recognition but, along with encounters with other patients around the same time, it opened me to powerful realizations about the clinical life. (274)

The emphasis here on the two women's similarities in terms of literacy, race, class, and gender is elided as inconsequential to the moment of recognition; for Charon, this moment would have happened anyway. My own work demonstrates that this moment inevitably would not have happened had her client been differently situated. For instance, diabetes might have had a different marker for a Black or Latinx person for whom diabetes is a prominent community condition; for women and men who, because of conditions of poverty, lack access to particular kinds of food and exercise, are seen as more deserving of diabetes; for the ESOL speaker or immigrant who does not share the same literacy skills (not just in terms of actual vocabulary but in the style and framework of the notes). While her client in this case is appreciative of her notes, Charon is unaware of how much this appreciation is dependent on the political economy of stigma.

Because narrative medicine as a brand works as one more piece of expertise-building, other medical practitioners are quickly attaching themselves to this brand and publishing more practical textbooks around incorporating narrative medicine into everyday medical practice. In 2016 Springer International released a book-length treatment, written by an Italy-based practitioner with years of international fellowships and service, Maria Giulia Marini. In this textbook, Marini argues for the inclusion of narrative medicine within evidence-based medicine and provides a background history of each (drawing deeply from Charon's 2008 text). Split into eleven chapters, the final "chapter" consisting of over thirty pages of "patient" narratives divided by diagnosis with no context for where or how these stories were captured, the book focuses on how narrative can be used by medical practitioners. Here is the irony; while Charon argues that narrative medicine can be one way to counter the practice of eight-minute visits with practitioners and thus create a more holistic practice of health care and healing, in order to argue its validity to mainstream medical practice, Marini argues that NM can make practitioners more efficient, reversing the initial impetus of the practice.

Marini's argument comes to its synthesis in her seventh chapter, "Bridging the Gap between Personalization of Care and Research" (59–69). Evidence-based medicine, according to Marini's definition and history, emerges in the 1970s to focus on population-based medicine as opposed to individual care; as a result, there is an emphasis in evidence-based practice on statistics and a devaluation of individualized narratives (1–5). Marini cites 2014 research that demonstrates more than half of physicians believe EBM is failing despite its widespread use in North America and Europe (4–6). For Marini, narrative medicine offers a cure for this practice; she does not, however, ask us to abandon evidence-based medicine but instead to incorporate NM into EBM (59–69). As Marini writes in her chapter 7 opening, "Narrative Medicine, despite the differing philosophical issues distinguishing it from EBM, can itself produce 'metrics' and numbers—tools that are valid for fast decision-making" (59). Marini proposes that new technologies can now support an analysis of narrative text, producing the kind of quantitative data used by EBM from subjective, qualitative data (59–60). Marini discusses her own work collecting patient stories to answer such questions as "How and when does solidity between family members develop in the unfolding of a chronic disease?" and "How much effort goes into managing a chronic disabling illness?" (61). As a humanities scholar, I am quick to question how one might "measure" the "solidity" of a relationship or the "effort" of managing a disease. Yet Marini provides a solution, using the software, NVivo, which can decipher the type of narrative by analyzing the length of sentences and the choice and repetition of words, providing three categories for stories: "disease-centred stories, illness-centred stories and between disease and illness-centred stories" (63). With this practice, storytelling can become quantified and usable for clinicians (62–64). Left out of this analysis are the particularities of illness, the context of power dynamics, and most importantly for my research interventions, attention to disparate literacy practices that fail to attend to how and why patients might deplore narrative strategies in the first place. No attention is paid to histories of abuse and the negation of privacy; instead, this practice of collecting stories and using software for interpretation increases the likelihood of administrative violence toward those marginalized by systems of racism, classism, sexism, homophobia, and ableism.

In her ninth chapter, Marini reinforces the need to introduce NM into EBM by arguing that the practice will make medical practitioners less likely to make mistakes in care, decreasing the overall cost of care (81–87). In this chapter, Marini focuses on those "decision-makers" and health-care economists who provide the data that informs health insurance companies which kinds of treatments are the most cost-effective. As opposed to asking the health insurance industry to make reforms to their profit-based model of care, Marini proposes that NM be used to support the industry's status quo (84–85). For Marini, narrative can be used to avoid "defensive" medicine and move toward preventive medicine. While I do not disagree that preventive medicine can be important (funding nutritious food, access accommodations, yoga classes), prevention itself is understood through practices of ableism: who is already "healthy" can participate in practices to sustain their health; who is not is somehow at fault for not participating in the "correct" preventive activities. While Marini does argue that preventive medicine is not profit-making in the way that pharmaceutical medicine is, she also argues that this is cost saving; the value in the narrative is one that can be attached to monetary value.

This understanding of narrative coincides with Margrit Shildrick's contention that debility itself represents intrinsic profitability under neoliberalism. "Where capital has historically relied on a population that through its labor necessarily becomes debilitated, the newer model of understanding represents the intrinsic profitability of debility itself," Shildrick (2015, 10–11) writes, referencing Jasbir Puar's work that distinguishes between disability as a Western concept and debility as it reflects globalized systems of capital and labor (11). "At the most fundamental level, it is in the interests of neo-liberalism to produce and sustain bodies as debilitated and therefore susceptible to a range of market commodities that hold out the promise of therapeutic interventions into the relative failures of physical, cognitive, and affective embodiment" (11).

While Shildrick is writing here about the individual bodies in need of constant therapeutic intervention because of neoliberal models of the always-striving-for-healthy self, I want to propose that narrative medicine works as a neoliberal therapeutic intervention on two levels: first, as a product for patient-clients to consume as another kind of wellness specialty; second, as a therapeutic corrective to capital "M" Medicine itself. To this last point, Medicine has been critiqued, under the model of the insurance industry, for not providing patient-centered care; what Marini does with her text on narrative medicine is to offer narrative medicine as a therapy for Medicine itself, a way to "treat" medicine so that it may continue to function within the efficiency framework while presenting a new, ever-necessary product to consumers. As Shildrick reminds us, "In the current politico-economic climate, to be debilitated does not place one outside societal or even individual norms; there is no bounded category to be othered" (11–12). Therefore, within the political economy of stigma, the debilitated consumer-patient becomes the sought-after client, whose stories themselves can be treated as a product, the process represented as a treatment in and of itself. Through this process Medicine, previously a broken system in need of rehabilitation, becomes cured. Put another way, narrative medicine becomes a rehabilitative tool for the medical industrial complex, while garnering the benefits of turning patient narratives into circulated product. This, in turn, works to support what feminist disability studies scholar Julie Elman terms *rehabilitative citizenship,* a form of citizenship rooted in emotional or cultural attachment that emerges in the intimate publics of the late twentieth century (6–7).[8] In fact, I would argue that the interest in and success of medical narrative and the political economy of stigma in which these narratives circulate is a direct effect of rehabilitative citizenship. If, in Elman's formulation, to become rehabilitative is to become a good citizen, then what narrative medicine does is resituate the effects of structural injustice as individual ailments to be eradicated through the negation of privacy for multiply marginalized people—relinquish privacy in order to be a good citizen.

Narrative medicine is marketed as the cure for neoliberal medicine while, in effect, it circulates narrative as a product for medical consumption. As a solution for commodifying patient stories, Lisa Diedrich suggests reading as "a witnessing of impossibility" (2007, 130). Diedrich calls us to formulate an "ethics of failure: that is, an ethics that emerges out of, or along with, an expe-

---

8. This process of rehabilitating medicine, or narrative medicine as a rehabilitative product for the medical industrial complex, is inspired by the arguments that feminist disability studies scholar Julie Elman makes about afterschool teen dramas in the 1970s and 1980s, which she terms "rehabilitative edutainment" (1–7).

rience of failure, be it of the body, of (conventional and alternative) medicine, or of language" (148). In conversation with Olivia Banner's and Lisa Diedrich's work, I understand that memoir offers us an opportunity to read for a failure of structures—medical, educational, political. My argument, however, is slightly different: while Banner and Diedrich argue that we can read for an understanding of structural oppression, my work highlights how reading itself can be an act of oppression through narrative entitlement. Our reading is shaped through the political economy of stigma, our access to narrative an effect of our relationship to privacy as a product of privilege.

Narrative medicine is one more way in which the political economy of stigma functions, shaping author–reader reception and creating cultures of belonging. How, then, do we move forward? In part III, *Beyond the Parallel Chart,* I explore precisely this question.

PART III

BEYOND THE
PARALLEL CHART

CHAPTER 5

Work, Disclosure, and the HIV Origin Story

Why Work Matters: HIV Origin Stories
for Women Living with HIV

Work matters. When I began my first reading group, I asked each woman with whom I did an intake interview to tell me a bit about themselves. They always began with the story of how they became infected with HIV; this in and of itself was not surprising given the context of our meeting location (at a local ASO), the context of my research and the materials I used to recruit (asking for women living with HIV to participate in a reading group study), and the number of times they are asked for details of their infection by medical providers. What was surprising was how prominently for all women interviewed, even those who did not end up participating in the book group, they situated their experience of infection and diagnosis within their experience as workers. In other words, where they were working and how their workplace responded to their HIV were central in their HIV origin stories told to me. Coincidentally, all women I interviewed were also currently not working for formal wages. The material conditions that living with HIV changes—with the cost of medications, the limitations of the pre-existing conditions in receiving health insurance,[1] and medication side effects—have led all of my group

1. When the Affordable Care Act Passed in 2012, the elimination of health-care companies' pre-existing condition limitations significantly changed the experience of medical access for research participants. Private insurance companies can no longer discriminate against

participants living with HIV to have an ambivalent relationship with paid work. They see themselves as future workers as well as past workers whose careers were interrupted or transformed by HIV.

This relationship to formal work directly affected these research participants' understandings of themselves as nondisabled citizens. While the structure of work itself and what is available to participants at the intersection of race, class, and gender have worked together to create disabling conditions, the women in this study did not identify as disabled, primarily because they see themselves as able to participate in a paid labor economy. The reason for this has everything to do with claiming citizenship in a neoliberal economy that values paid labor. Doing so, they are resisting common racialized and gendered stereotypes circulating through the political economy of stigma, even while problematically reinforcing the ableist relationship between labor and citizenship.

The political economy of stigma relies on the intersection of ableism with racism, sexism, classism, and homophobia. In order to address how the political economy of stigma interacts with systems of oppression and privilege, we need to revisit Kimberlé Crenshaw's original work in intersectionality. Crenshaw begins theorizing intersectionality by looking at workplace discrimination cases where the law understands race and gender as mutually exclusive categories (139). For Crenshaw, single-axis analysis actually distorts Black women's experience (139–40). We can extend Crenshaw here to thinking about ableism and the law, understanding that the political economy of stigma works by obscuring the intersection of oppressions. In the emphasis on individual accommodation, and the contention of one's worthiness of such accommodation, group barriers of exclusion are obscured; one can access disability legal services in light of workplace discrimination if they, in fact, have a workplace; one's experience of themselves as disabled is radically contingent on their relationships to paid work. In the experiences of the women living with HIV with whom I worked, the very process by which they came to disclose their HIV was in the context of their jobs. Further, their relationship with author Catherine Wyatt-Morley, and her own disclosures of workplace discrimination, is what enabled their complex disclosures to me, as a researcher. Thus, in resisting the political economy of stigma, and the way it mediates author–reader relations, we were all able to question the foundations of the law, reinforcing Crenshaw's careful critique of single-axis analysis.

---

women for having HIV. This has been on the table once again in during the 2020 presidential election, during which I am revising this chapter.

Crenshaw theorizes that antidiscrimination law addresses the wrongness of using race and gender in decisions that would otherwise be neutral (151). This is not grounded in a bottom-up commitment to ending discrimination (151). Thus, antidiscrimination law addresses those who are privileged "but for" race or gender (151). This is also what disability law does. In her conclusions, Crenshaw argues that we need to expand both feminist theory and antiracist politics by "embracing the intersection" (166). Embracing the intersection is not about seeing individuals as discriminated against but about undermining the political economy of stigma, which obscures how labor is so central in one's negotiation of identity. Resisting the political economy of stigma, produced through author–reader relations, provides an opportunity for the women living with HIV in my reading group to develop a sophisticated political consciousness, central to which is the authors' relationships to work, their own work experience, and the process of HIV disclosure.[2]

In this chapter, I do a close reading and narrative analysis of my first book-group participants' negotiation with material labor, capturing as much of their own voices as possible as they recount experiences of workplace discrimination due to HIV. I then turn to disability legal theory and Black feminist legal theory to theorize the significance of labor, and one's ability to work, in the construction of disability discrimination and the internalization of ableism. Doing so, I question the dominant binary of internalized ableism versus externalized resistance. Ultimately, I question the utility of the Americans with Disability Act for women living with HIV, returning again to the availability of disability identification within the political economy of stigma. I want to be clear that the availability of disability identification is neither positive nor negative but merely an effect of the political economy of stigma produced through author–reader relations.

I first address the relationship that women living with HIV build with author Catherine Wyatt-Morley and how Wyatt-Morley's work enables group members to disclose their own HIV origin stories; second, I recount the HIV origin stories of three women living with HIV in my first reading group, demonstrating how central to each woman's narrative is her experience of work; third, I address AIDS service workers' disconnections from Wyatt-Morley's

---

2. Within disability studies, there is some reflection and theorization about disclosure and HIV. Achim Nowak wrote a particularly useful piece about the process of disclosing HIV status to employers and medical insurance companies, from his first diagnosis in the late 1980s through the early 2000s, questioning how and when disclosure of HIV status is necessary. For the women I worked with, their process of disclosing has some similarities to Nowak's experience but also opens up more questions about precarity and other welfare assistance programs. Chris Bell also writes about disclosure in relation to sexual partners, productively questioning notions of cultural responsibility and AIDS criminalization laws.

work and their own experience of becoming AIDS service workers. This chapter moves us beyond Charon's "parallel chart" and the practice of narrative medicine critiqued in part II because it captures the individual experiences of illness and diagnosis within larger structural and material contexts that highlight how the political economy of stigma obscures structural oppression.

Catherine's Disclosure as Closing Temporality

Catherine Wyatt-Morley's memoir was disliked by all but one member of my AIDS service worker reading group. Because Wyatt-Morley's memoir was so well received by my first reading group, the intensity of this negative reaction surprised me. Some members disliked it because of the style of writing; Wyatt-Morley writes in a journal style, inserting some poetry (by herself and by other women living with HIV) and some educational materials. As Diana, who has been in the AIDS activist movement since 1982, tells me, "I actually really liked her. I was taken by her plan and her story and all that. I just didn't want to read her diary" (10/27/2015). For Nick, who was born one year before Wyatt-Morley published her book and thus missed the entire early AIDS movement, the diary itself does not feel authentic: "I just feel like it was over-edited. That someone read this and changed everything she wrote and made it sound like'—but before he can finish his thought, another group member, Tony, says, "Isn't that the process of writing a book, though?" (10/27/2015). While this is one of the final books that we read together, this is the first time the group discusses the process of writing together and questions the role of the editor.

Adam, who "hated" the book and the tone because he thought it was too "Pollyanna" in relation to her Christian message, reflects on Wyatt-Morley's writing: "I think she probably wrote this way because when she started writing, she thought she was going to die. So, if I start my journal, write in it every day, at least there will be something left in it for my kids. For someone to benefit from. No matter at what point I die" (5/27/2015). Tony, who is male-bodied, the only person of color in the group, and the only avid reader of memoir before the group started, responds: "It's not just because it is easier for the writer to write that way. But I think that's for someone who she tried to reach as a reader, it's easier for them to read that way, too" (5/27/2015). Without explicitly saying so, Tony highlights the literacy disparities between many low-income Black women (the fastest-growing HIV population at the time Wyatt-Morley publishes her memoir) and the education level of the group.

The other negative complaints about Wyatt-Morley's memoir address her inability to leave her husband, who exposed Wyatt-Morley to HIV after having sexual relationships outside their marriage. The group diagnoses Wyatt-Morley as "codependent" and even comes to see her spiritual Christian practice as a part of this codependency. When I ask the group whether Wyatt-Morley may be speaking specifically to a Black audience about the Black church, the group responds by denying that there is a "race" issue in the memoir. As Adam, a White gay male psychiatric nurse, who has also gone to seminary and is active in a local Protestant church, tells the group, "I think it's not really a Black issue. It's more of a fundamentalist issue. White fundamentalists are the same way. Jesus tells me this. Jesus tells me that. Jesus in my heart. These are the kind of phraseology you would see with any fundamentalist" (5/27/2015). Adam goes on to explain that fundamentalists are "myopic" (5/27/2015). "That's where I would like divergences on her part. Get away from the Pollyanna view of God and really talk about spirituality," Adam concludes. What this conversation opens up is an opportunity for the group to talk about their own spiritual practices, some Christian and some not; none of them, however, make the connection between their own spiritual practice and their HIV work, a connection that Wyatt-Morley makes explicit throughout her text.

In my final interviews, almost everyone ranks Wyatt-Morley's memoir at the bottom of their lists. Tony is the only exception to the ASO worker group, arguing that Wyatt-Morley's memoir was "really good" and that he enjoyed all the memoirs that addressed racism in some way (12/11/2015). Most agree with Adam, who says, "It was good to read because it was historical, but we don't really have any patients like that anymore" (11/24/2015). This comment may resonate with the other members of the group because of the new emphasis on long-term living with HIV and the ASO's involvement with promoting the newly FDA-approved PrEP (Pre-Exposure Prophylactic). The atmosphere of this ASO is one of long-term care and optimism, making the experience of those in the 1990s feel long ago. Yet one of the main reasons why the women living with HIV that I worked with consistently circled back to Wyatt-Morley's work was that it enabled them to make direct connections to both workplace discrimination and medical discrimination in their own lives. In exploring these connections in the next section, my research participants living with HIV directly contradict Adam's assertion that "we just don't have patients like this anymore."

Judy: From Warehouse Labor to Community College

Adam and Judy do not know one another. None of the participants in my first reading group would have any way of knowing the participants in my second given that the groups take place in different cities with connections to different AIDS service organizations. Yet Judy's story is not dissimilar to some that Adam would encounter in his own work. And for Judy, her experiences of work and discrimination are central to her understanding of herself as an HIV survivor.

When Judy was diagnosed in the mid-1990s, she had been working in a warehouse in the Southeast US. The day following her diagnosis, Judy went to work. "I didn't miss. I had a job," she recounts to me in our first meeting, the meeting where I ask her to tell me about her experience with HIV (8/23/2012). "I was working in a warehouse, trying to support my family. My kids, they were teenagers. And I had to go to work. Like there wasn't nothing to it" (8/23/2012). In Judy's HIV story, work remains the central touchstone for conveying how HIV became a normalized aspect of her daily life. Eventually, the job at the warehouse became too much for Judy, based in part on a work-related injury. "And I end up, I relocated here [our current city] it started getting difficult for, you know, I was doing warehouse work and I was so speeding and constantly on the line and I started, I couldn't, I started slowing and I just couldn't keep up" (8/23/2012). Judy explains the pinched nerve in her back, her supervisor's insistence that an MRI would cost her $1,000 through the company's worker's compensation program, and her longer-term ignoring of the issue. "I was like, I'll be alright" (8/23/2012). At this time, Judy also experienced HIV stigma in the workplace, a story that emerges not in our first meeting but later, in connection to Catherine Wyatt-Morley's memoir:

> Just because she was infected in 1994 and she couldn't tell her boss. I can relate to that. I couldn't. I was working in a company, too. She was working in a plant. I was working in a warehouse. I couldn't tell. I felt like if I told my boss, he would find a reason to let me go. I couldn't afford at that time to risk losing my job. I had a family to take care of. And the type of work I was doing, he would have found a way to replace me. (11/1/2012)

Judy recounts rumors about other people becoming ill and being let go: "lawsuits going on up there and everything" (11/1/2012). Because of the low-skilled qualifications for Judy's work in the warehouse, she was replaceable, which makes both disclosure and accommodation inaccessible to her. When I mention that her experience of withholding HIV sounds scary, she reflects on further stigma:

> Yah, it was real scary. And then I hear people, they be talking, I hear people. There be one gay guy working and we were having Thanksgiving, and I heard

somebody say, "I know he didn't touch those greens. I know he didn't put his hands in there" and I say "Lord, have mercy!" That affected me. I'm like, he ain't even, he's just gay. They know this but if I was to tell them mine, if everybody knew about it or whatever, they want everybody to pitch in and bring food and you think they would want to eat after me? I heard them talk about him. I'm like, "Lord Jesus, I ain't going to be able to stay here much longer." I didn't like the way they were talking. I have to come in sick. Don't feel good. Fatigued. I had to pretend. I didn't know what was hitting me. But I had to work. I had to support my family. The fatigue was hitting me. I would rest in breaks. It was nine and a half hours a day and in between time, at lunch, I would take a nap. (11/1/2012)

Judy first recounts the stigma associated with sexuality and HIV but then remembers the physical effects of her HIV. In fact, in many of our conversations, for Judy the HIV doesn't become physical until the stigma itself is unpacked for discussion in our reading groups. In our initial interview, Judy's experience with HIV does not factor in to her reason for leaving her warehouse work and relocating, attributing her move to her work-related back injury. But in the context of our reading group discussion, and Wyatt-Morley's experience with work-related discrimination in a similar workplace, similar region, and same period, Judy accesses the embodiment of her early HIV experience. This fatigue could very well be part of her reason to leave her strenuous warehouse work.

Judy moved to our current city because her daughter had already relocated here. Judy had trouble finding work because of her physical pain, and although her husband followed her in the relocation, she remained the primary wage earner in her relationship. It was not until she was able to separate from her husband, who was dealing drugs, that she began to understand HIV as a central part of her life. In essence, her physical disability provided separation from warehouse work, giving her the time and energy to address her HIV status, which had, up until then, not disrupted her work. Because HIV was unable to disrupt her daily life initially, it remained unaddressed. Judy continues reflecting on her relocation, a narrative she intersperses with relationship and family experiences—the story she tells follows no direct linear path:

My worker I have here, she got me on disability. It took me three years to get that. They didn't want to give it to me then. Basically, I got, not a pinched nerve but a sort of like, I got a disk that got replaced. Like an old Ford. When I moved here in 03, I got this pain. I think it's related to the job I had. [. . .] I've been seeing a pain specialist. It's three discs out of place. Not just out of

> place. They're deteriorating. Joint disease or whatever. That's a disease, okay?
> Along with the HIV. It's been a process. (8/23/2012)

Here Judy, for the first time, claims HIV as a disease, but notably only in the context of another disease. As she speaks she is also seeking affirmation that I believe she is speaking from a medical truth, a habit that may come from having to "prove" her pain and disability in the context of disability assistance. It is also interesting that Judy compares her body to a machine, a practical, working Ford, understanding her body as utilitarian. I ask, "So is it the back pain that you are able to get on Social Security?" "More so than the HIV," she responds. "The HIV it was like, well, your CD4 count is this and your viral load is this, and you know, you ain't in the AIDS stage, of course, I wasn't" (8/12/2012). For Judy, and women like Judy, the HIV alone is not enough to qualify for disability assistance; Judy meets disability qualification because of her work-related chronic pain and her HIV status. HIV can only become disability when it disrupts one's ability to participate in the formal labor economy.

Judy is now enrolled in a program designed to find part-time work for people on disability. Yet Judy's former work experience, and corresponding class background, makes it nearly impossible for her to find work: "My experience has got me limited because education today requires computer skills. Some jobs I would love to have, sitting in an office, answering phones, you know, doing the computer from time to time, but you know, you have to have that experience" (8/23/2012). Over the course of the nine months that Judy and I got to know each other, Judy enrolled in a local community college with the initial intention of building her computer skills. We met in July 2012, and in January, at our first group meeting after the holidays, Judy reflects on her experience in college: "I didn't know that this [Addiction Studies] was going to be what I major in," Judy laughs, recounting her week's experience to the group (1/17/2013).

> Actually, I didn't. I didn't come to realize it until I was in the Admissions Office, and I had the areas broken down because my main focus going in there was to take up computers, to have computer knowledge. So, computer science was a major and they broke it down "this is what you would be doing, all this office work," and I was like, "I don't think this is what I want." And I mentioned counseling. (1/17/2013)

As Judy's first semester of school continues, she remains the most consistent book group attendee. She frequently talks with me, before the other participants arrive, about her challenges with reading, writing, and commuting to school. "When you take a bus, it's different, with a condition like mine," Judy tells me in the middle of flu season (1/24/2013). Susceptibility to viruses, and their ability to fight off something like the flu, continues to be a fear for the women in my group.

While Judy is only attending school "part time," her workload with two classes is still forty hours a week. This is a direct reflection of the intersection of HIV and class background, where, despite her finishing high school, her education has not prepared her for the current job market. Judy did complete her semester but she unenrolled in her disability work program. In our final interview, Judy was still enrolled in school and on Social Security. I asked Judy whether she saw herself as a person with disability; the disability identity continued to remain unavailable to her (3/26/2013).

I explained to Judy that the law, because of her HIV status, allows her to access disability resources. She responded firmly:

> Well the law may say that, but the law is going to give you a sure enough time accessing disability because of the experience it took me! I became disability [sic] not because of my HIV actually but because of the other condition. My back condition. If it was left up to the HIV, I probably wouldn't get it. It took me three years to get it! Because of the HIV and that combined together, it was looked at. (3/26/2013)

Here, Judy does claim disability as identity, "I became disability," but only in the context of accessing these resources, resources that become available because of her multiple physical conditions.

Judy doesn't mention in the context of work and disability her addiction recovery; at the time of our first meeting, she had been sober eight months (8/23/2012). While Judy does understand her addiction as a disease, she never relates it to disrupting her work. Again, in the context of Catherine Wyatt-Morley's memoir, I get a brief insight about the relationship between addiction and work in Judy's life (11/1/2012). Morley writes of her husband's alcoholism, the primary reason the two eventually get divorced. Judy explains to the group how she doesn't agree with Morley's decision to divorce because "he was functional, he was going to work" (11/1/2012). Judy never mentions her own addiction disrupting her ability to work; thus, while it is a disease, it doesn't enter the disability framework that she outlines for herself. Ironically, addiction recovery is the reason she wants to return to work as a counselor. She no longer wants to work simply for a paycheck, especially without having children or a husband at home to support. Judy is satisfied remaining on her Social Security so that she can continue school. She is not the only group member whose philosophies of work, and what kinds of labor she is willing to participate in, change in the course of the reading group and in relation to her own sophisticated political consciousness.

Elizabeth: From Informal Caregiver to the Labor of Self-Care

When I first met Elizabeth, she had only had her HIV diagnosis for two years, being the most recently diagnosed woman in the group (8/23/2012). A mother and grandmother, she had been the primary wage earner and caregiver for her family; at the time of her diagnosis, she no longer had kids at home. I asked about her work history at the time of her diagnosis. "A few years prior to that [HIV diagnosis], I had gotten into a car accident that really messed up my back. So, I was dealing with that. So, when I was going to the doctors and everything, I wasn't able to work and I was waiting on my disability. I didn't want to go on disability" (8/23/2012). Throughout our getting to know one another, Elizabeth always emphasized wanting to go back to work, as I analyzed in chapter 1. Elizabeth understood her disability assistance as only temporary; it was also not directly connected to her HIV status.

Of all three participants, Elizabeth provided the shortest initial interview, discussing her interest in reading more than her relationship to HIV or work. In our first group meeting, however, Elizabeth opened up more after Judy and Mary shared their experiences. While Elizabeth was on disability because of her car accident, she also mentions, as part of her HIV origin story, a long-term boyfriend who was unfaithful and abusive (she mentions casually in our last session "since my stabbing incident" and I don't ask for more details though I have noticed the scar in the upper right of her chest) (10/25/2012). This isolation and abuse may have contributed to her inability to work. She also mentions in the context of writing—when we are having a discussion about what it might be like to write our own memoirs—how physically difficult writing can be for her. "I have a disability as far as a paralysis in my hand from a stroke that I had. So, I sit at a computer or typewriter and type something out, I have to do in, you know, my own little way to try to keep up, you know? And, like, I thought it was so cool that they came out with this software that puts out your words on the screen, you can look at it" (1/17/2013). In the context of paid labor, Elizabeth consistently evaluates her own physical limitations, at times identifying as a person with disability, at other times only as a person *on* disability. During our group sessions, however, she does not actually connect her disability to her HIV.

At the same time, Elizabeth does connect her HIV to a change in self-esteem; this change affects what she views as possible in her work life. "'Cause I thought it was, I really felt when I first got my diagnosis back, that it was the end of the world. I was never going to do anything to try to make up for it or to compensate, you know what I mean? But today I feel like I've got so much more, so much more I want to do. And I've got a chance to do it" (2/7/2013). Elizabeth relates this change in her self-esteem partly to reading our group's HIV memoirs over the holidays and partly to making a commitment to therapy provided by the HIV center where we meet. But most importantly, she connects this shift in her self-understanding to her ability to draw boundaries. "I've always been in and out and in and out and I never really stayed in it, you know?" Elizabeth begins, tracing her experience with one-on-one counseling:

> This is the first time I have constantly stayed in counseling and gone through it, put the work in and really learned a lot about myself—in over 25 years. I knew, after being diagnosed, I knew a lot of things had to change, a lot of things were going to change, whether I wanted them to or not, all right? And in order for me to be able to deal with that change, I had to do some work of my own, you know? I've become more confident. I have more self-respect, self-esteem, than I ever had growing up! (2/7/2013)

While a few months into our book group, Elizabeth begins to see herself wanting to go back to work, the financial issues related to forgoing disability are too daunting: "I've thought about it because if I did go back to work, you know, doctors, am I going to be able to afford doctors, that type of thing. The financial issue of it, that standpoint" (1/17/2013). Elizabeth confides in the group her hesitations after we have been talking about the advocacy work of one of our memoirists, Regan Hoffman, former editor of the HIV magazine *POZ*. In connection to reading Hoffman, Elizabeth tells the group of her plans for work. It is in the context of this conversation that I learn that Elizabeth, before her accident, worked as a medical assistant. She tells me of her interest in getting back into that labor market.

> ELIZABETH: I have decided that I want to go back to school to be retrained. Because, I guess, lately, I've just been seeing I've gotta, I've outgrown my little four walls I've gotten into right now and I got to have more and I want to be a little better prepared and comfortable.
>
> A: So, what does it mean? To go back to school for you?
>
> ELIZABETH: To be retrained. I already found what school I want to go to. I chose that because they have the curriculum I'm looking for. Which is a growing field already. And I think, um, as I do that, I'll also be able

to, you know, get more involved into this HIV study thing and maybe branch out. You know what I'm saying? So, I'll have a specific area that I want to go into once I get done.

A: And you think you will figure out how to make your job HIV-related in the end?

ELIZABETH: That's right. Because I want to, um, this is something that crossed my mind. This is what I want. The last couple of years, I've been going through this, in and out of doctor's offices, different types of doctors' offices, and you get familiar with the scene. [The group, including K., laughs]. [. . .] And that's what has really gotten me like, "We need more people." (1/17/2013)

Elizabeth has always been an informal caregiver within her family and friend community but, upon the suggestion of a friend that she go to nursing school, she resisted. "Because I get too attached, you know what I'm saying," and she recounts her experience of the past few weeks arranging hospice care for her neighbor (1/17/2013). Elizabeth's boundaries with the kind of work she is willing to do shift in our time together; this is another demonstration of how resisting the political economy of stigma produces an author–reader relationship that makes room for Elizabeth to develop a sophisticated political consciousness. Disability studies scholar Fiona Kumari Campbell has written astutely about how one must negotiate able-bodied norms in order to access legal resources (30–36). This is because disability is understood in the law as deficiency; this deficiency is assumed by ableist culture; thus, in order to access the law, disabled people must embrace disability as a negative state (36). The law creates dissonance between official and private realities. Both Judy and Elizabeth express this dissonance; both women are on disability but neither identify as having a disability, at least not as a stable identity or as an identity connected to their HIV. Through the political economy of stigma, the memoir industry produces reader–author relationships that enhance the dissonance between official and private realities, but for some, reading in resistance to the political economy of stigma is what provides room for the development of a political consciousness.[3]

---

3. Ruth Colker, a disability legal theorist, proposes one way to address this dissonance created by the law; for Colker, we should measure equality from an antisubordination perspective (2009, 1). In an antisubordination model, it is a lack of power, and not difference itself, that is the problem. Colker proposes a statistical significance approach to disability and the law (62). This approach will cover Americans with some sort of measurable impairment (vision, hearing) whose ability falls two standards deviations below the mean, while also covering those with impairments that cannot be measured. Additionally, we need to keep in mind that the two standard deviations below the mean should be considered the floor of coverage, not the ceiling

Mary's Negotiations:
From Businesswoman to Plaintiff

Mary, at thirty-five, is the youngest of the participants in my group. She's also never been married and never had children. She was working on commission, selling insurance for a small company at the time of her HIV diagnosis. When we first met, she was unemployed, with a discrimination lawsuit under investigation (10/22/2012). When I asked her about her experience with HIV, she spoke candidly about her work experience, HIV becoming prominent in her life because of workplace discrimination:

> Well, I've always been one hundred percent commission. So, my job depends on my personality, where you have to have one hundred and twenty percent work ethic, when that's how your life is maintained. I don't have children. I went for money money money. I went for the highest-paying job I could find. I was with them two or three years before I was diagnosed. So, I'm with this company and there are only two women. Of course. So, I'm one of their top producers. They are Christian-based they say. (11/1/2012)

Mary pauses here and emphasizes the Christian-identity of the company, extending the "ay" sound of *say* and raising her voice for effect. She tells me that the company president is an ordained minister and that they regularly pray at staff meetings. Mary identifies herself as a Christian and feels comfortable with this company practice. It is also important for Mary that she is one of only two women, that she is a top salesperson in a company dominated by men. This combination of her gender identity and success in business is a continual point of pride and self-esteem for Mary; being a businesswoman is a theme she raises many times over the course of our nine months getting to know one another.

Mary was at work when she received confirmation of her HIV test results from her doctor. Because she was in a meeting at the time, and stepped out

---

(62). Colker's emphasis on measurement actually does little to rectify the subordination of disability. This proposal also excludes unmeasurable disabilities: How much HIV does one have to have in order to qualify for discrimination coverage? If an employer discriminates against you for living with HIV, does the discrimination not count if your viral load is below 500? What about the compounding of multiple conditions? While Colker does address the problems with unmeasurable conditions such as mental illness, she argues that courts should be able to "try on" different definitions of disability to see what works—the goal being to cover those who need it—she never addresses the problem of the ableism of the law itself (63). How would a law work that addresses a fluid identification with disability, one that resists measuring from some sort of "norm"?

to take the phone call, she felt compelled to tell her boss and his son, her co-worker. "And we immediately called his father, who anointed me and prayed for me." A week later, after Mary won a sales competition (in competition with 300 employees) and was invited to travel with her supervisor a few hours away for the awards ceremony, she felt confident to ask for some accommodations:

> So, I'm like, listen. Right now, I am still in shock. And I don't know how I'm going to react. I don't know how I'm going to feel. I do know that I am going to need time to process this. I don't want to work as much. I want to be closer to my family. At that time, I had been driving out to L. every day, you know, a two-hour drive back and forth every day. I was just, like, I need to cut back on work. I've worked my ass off. This is something tragic. I don't know how to understand it yet. They of course prayed with me. I left feeling like, okay, this is going to be cool. (11/1/2012)

Less than a week after that encounter, Mary was given a sales route into a nearby state, a route that required three- to four-hour drives each way. "I mean, basically, he took a stereotype and he knew darn well what he was doing [. . .] He knew I had a strong enough personality that I would come in one day and say fuck off [laughing] and I did. Probably a month or two into it" (11/1/2012). There are several reasons I can hypothesize that Mary was able to feel comfortable leaving her job in a way that Judy was not. Mary grew up in a middle-class family; her father is business owner himself; and when her job search in the following months turned up more HIV-related discrimination (I'll return to this in a moment), she knew she was able to work for her father's contracting company. She was also financially secure, with savings and retirement, at the time of her diagnosis. She had never experienced racial discrimination in the workplace, as a White woman, though she does allude to sexism when she emphasizes her experience as one of only a few women in a 300-person company. Mary also holds a bachelor's degree in business, which provides her job market qualifications the other participants in my group do not have. Finally, Mary's brother is an attorney, which gives her familiarity with the law and access to free legal consultation; when I ask her, however, about whether she is filing for disability discrimination, she is unaware that HIV is a protected status.

After leaving her job and taking a few months off to process her HIV status, Mary began interviewing for new sales positions. Within a few weeks of interviewing, Mary received a job offer from a new company.

> The last day he was like, Mary, everything about you, I love but I can tell there is a wall. There's something wrong with you. And I was like, "Well, there are

personal things in my life that I don't want to talk about," and he was like, "You have to tell me. This is my business, my baby. I need to know if anything is in our way. You can tell me. It's not going to make a difference." You know, again, and I told him. So, you know, I was composed, I didn't need his pity, or his "I'm sorry" or his hug. I told him, he acted like he understood what it was; he was like, "Thank you, I could tell something was in the way." So, he's like "I'll speak to you soon," and I walked out the door and never heard from him. Never got a call saying, "No thank you, we went with someone else." (11/1/2012)

Mary recounts this as the second time she experienced workplace discrimination as a result of disclosing her HIV status. When Mary had trouble finding sales positions, she went to work at her father's company, where she experienced an accident that left her with chronic back pain. After months on bed rest, Mary went to work part-time for a sales company, operating inbound phone calls, where she again experienced discrimination, this time from her younger co-workers. "They saw me as this businesswoman, whose family is well off, why is she working a part-time job at ten bucks an hour? And in reality, they didn't know it was because I was disabled. And I was. It wasn't my HIV. It was that fall" (11/1/2012). Here, Mary briefly claims a disability identity, but like Judy and Elizabeth, she distinguishes between her disability and her HIV. She recounts that she began missing work because of chronic sinus infections, "and of course they'd last three weeks; with the HIV, they would take forever to heal" (11/1/2012). Mary filed for leave under the Family Medical Leave Act. In Mary's following account, it is because of her HIV that Human Resources "set me up, got me out the door" (11/1/2012):

> After FMLA, anytime I was absent, it was because of my sinus. Or my back. I just wasn't feeling well. But then they saw my HIV status. I'm a year and a half into it. Instead of back-dating for the other instances, like they should have (I just found this out), they fired me because one day I actually came into work seven minutes late. They were just looking for a reason. And of course, they hadn't taken off those occurrences from a year ago, which I wasn't aware of. (11/1/2012)

Mary, with the assistance of her brother, filed a workers' compensation suit. When Mary's attorney held initial meetings with her workplace attorneys, more HIV discrimination took place. "I wasn't at the table," Mary recounts, "but I have it in writing. The attorneys came in and to my attorney they said, before we even got started, 'We've gone back through all of her medical records, she has AIDS. We're not paying her a dollar'" (11/1/2012). Following Mary's recounting of this incident, Judy and Mary began to talk with one another in quick succession. Elizabeth was not present for this particular reading group session.

> JUDY: That's hurtful. That's hurtful.
> MARY: I know. I cried.
> JUDY: Especially because they went to AIDS. I don't got AIDS.
> MARY: I know. I'm really sensitive about that.
> JUDY: I'm real sensitive about that!
> MARY: I have that in writing. That means in court, in trial, to the jurors, I'm beating that until the horse is dead!
> JUDY: I'm really sensitive about that because I experienced that with my pain specialist. They said I had AIDS. (11/1/2012)

The distinction between HIV and AIDS that both Mary and Judy are sensitive to is, perhaps, a distinction between illness and a medical condition; disability and a medical condition. Both women understand AIDS as a marker of decreased life expectancy and a limit to their long-term goals. Because of stigma, and what Mary and Judy both term "stupid ignorance," HIV becomes disabling.

Mary's case went to trial a few months into our reading group, not resulting in Mary's favor. I asked Mary, gently, whether she wanted to talk about it, but she was adamant: "I don't need to talk about my shit. It's not worth it" (3/07/2013). Then she changed the subject to Judy's recent dating. In our last book group meeting, when all three participants were together and talking informally about their weeks, Mary mentioned her court case again. "This week really hasn't been much about HIV—it's really just everything else. Job. Work. Finances. The workman's comp case. Nothing related to HIV this week" (3/07/2013). In the beginning, for Mary, the workers' compensation case had to do with disability discrimination, a back condition and a sinus condition that were both complicated by her weakened immune system; conditions that, in the context of the case, were disconnected from HIV. When her HIV came up between her attorneys, as a reason to deny her compensation, Mary was willing to draw upon her HIV discrimination to make a compensation claim. At the close of her case, she once again understood it as "not about HIV." Here, Mary demonstrates how she moves in and out of HIV identification, doing so in tension with and opposition to disability identification.

Political theorist Deborah Stone, in her 1984 book *The Disabled State*, traces how disability becomes an administrative category through the Social Security Administration, in the years before the ADA was passed (25–89).

Disability as an administrative category creates a boundary between work and need-based distributive systems (20–25): the definition of disability is the boundary (25). From the earliest origins of the category, those with chronic sickness were debated for inclusion precisely because their ability to work was unpredictable (41–44). The idea that the chronically sick were either waiting to be cured or somehow falsifying their claims of inability was foundational to how disability as an administrative category was legally conceptualized in Europe and the US. Stone's work is instructive but does not tell us how one relates to the administrative categories. She also does not interrogate how racial and gender discrimination interact with administrating disability claims. Legal and cultural studies scholar Fiona Kumari Campbell helps explain how and why Mary's resistance to identifying with disability happens as a result of legal systems.[4] Campbell draws on Fanon to understand how claiming a disability label in order to gain access does not mean that an individual believes they are disabled (26). These processes of claiming a disability when disability is viewed in ableist culture as negative can lead to an ongoing state of ambivalence (27–29). This ambivalence is precisely what I witnessed in my first conversations with the participants in my research group. When Mary, for instance, wants to highlight HIV discrimination in a workers' compensation case, but then is adamant about never using disability resources because she associates those resources with deteriorating health, she exhibits this ambivalence that Campbell describes.

At the close of our reading group and final interview, Mary was piecing together income from two part-time positions. I asked explicitly whether she saw HIV as a part of her identity. "I mean, it is when it comes to relationships, like my hair is brown, but I just don't know" (4/01/2013). She also asserted that HIV was not at the forefront of her identity, even though she had recently become detectable. When I asked whether she thought she would ever draw on disability resources because of her HIV, she exclaimed, animatedly, "I hope not! I don't want to! As far as I know, the medicines are going to keep me where I am right now!" (4/01/2013). I also asked whether, if there were a group in her church (since she is a devoted church member) for women with illness or disability, she would see herself as a part of it. "My life is rough," she said. "So definitely I see myself as a part of a group for support, recovery, what have you. HIV would be one of the many things that I am struggling with.

---

4. Although Campbell is an Australian scholar, her case study throughout the book is based on legal constructions in the US (primarily, the ADA and the Revised ADA) and its exportations to Western Europe and the UK. For these reasons, because her theorizing is rooted in American legal scholarship, her insights are useful for my project. Her ideas also build on the scholarship of Ruth Colker and Tobin Siebers.

But you know, it's just as equal as being poor and having this horrible injury from work and my house flooding. I mean, they are all equal!" (4/01/2013). Here, too, Mary moves in and out of disability identification, seeing herself as part of a group but also not wanting to draw on resources available (sometimes) to that group. HIV becomes synonymous with other kinds of struggles, an entanglement that highlights the complicated oppressions upon which the political economy of stigma thrives.

In their 2001 co-written article, Jennifer Pokempner and Dorothy Roberts trace the specific relationship between poverty and disability that Mary highlights above (1). We have a social insurance model for disability where the disabled are considered deserving (1). In contrast, the poor are blamed for failing to work (1). Disability benefits programs recognize that disability can cause poverty, but they don't look at how poverty can cause disability (1). For Mary, Elizabeth, and Judy, this perceived dichotomy is ever-present, affecting how they understand themselves in relation to the formal labor economy. For Elizabeth and Judy, who both come from working-class and working-poor backgrounds, poverty certainly affected the jobs available to them, which required repetitive physical tasks causing physical impairments that complicated their medical and workplace negotiations with HIV. Mary, as a White, college-educated woman, held an expectation for a certain kind of middle-class job, working for a small private company where workplace protections from disability discrimination were assumed. This assumption left her disappointed and angry when she became the target of discrimination. All three women are constantly negotiating the stigma of being unemployed and "undeserving" of benefits as poor people with the stigma of being disabled, deserving of benefits but presumed incapable of formal work. For Pokempner and Roberts, the dichotomy between disability and poverty is false. Because state responses to both poverty and disability are based on wage labor, exclusion and inequality are created by both having a similar relationship to power structures (1). Thus, we need systems of social support that address both disability and poverty together (3). I would go further to suggest that this system that creates this dichotomy between deserving and undeserving citizens, between disabled and poor, is reinforced by the political economy of stigma. For example, the group of ASO workers with whom I worked did not recognize this system of deserving and underserving bifurcation. This is an effect of the political economy of stigma. We know this because they called the recognition of its significance "historical" in the work of Wyatt-Morley. I worry about the invisibility of this power enacted through the political economy of stigma for those in medical positions of power. How can we heighten this visibility, read against the political economy of stigma?

Without heightening the visibility of these systems, we risk reinforcing the divide between deserving (disabled) and undeserving (poor) citizens. In Pokempner and Roberts's analysis, assistance for disability is premised on the idea that disability is outside the individual and thus beyond the individual's control; they are excused from the labor force (3). In contrast, the poor's need is considered their own fault (9). Although the ADA addresses social norms, it does not require economic and social structural change that would address poverty (i.e., we make adjustments as long as they are not too costly; 9). Similarly, addressing disability must be embedded in bigger antipoverty initiatives (9). Sociologist Celeste Watkins-Hayes notes that the Ryan White Act serves as a gold standard for addressing the overlapping needs of social and systemic change by providing not just access to medications but access to housing, transportation, complex medical care, and employment (178–203). And yet, despite the Ryan White Act's success, there is a move today to eliminate the larger social safety net for HIV in favor of the "test-and-treat revolution," once again disconnecting disability/medical need from poverty (178–203). By obscuring these systems of power that create a dichotomy between the poor and the disabled, the political economy of stigma reinforces as necessity harmful policy initiatives that view HIV clients as "noncompliant" and "troublesome," leading to the withholding of immediate medical care (medications) and the entrenchment of poverty.

In the next chapter, I explore the effects of the political economy of stigma's obscuration of power through the experience of administrative violence for women living with HIV. Ultimately, I propose that women living with HIV, as a result of the daily negotiation of administrative violence, provide a new practice for reading disability narrative.

CHAPTER 6

Power, Resistance, and Differential Reading Practices

When I began this project, I was surprised by how much the women living with HIV in my first group had a mobile identification with disability; Judy, Elizabeth, and Mary all varied in their relationships with a disability identification despite accessing disability-related services. They understood disability as a regulatory system of power and, thus, moved in and out of their relationship to it. One of the places where I saw this mobile identification most prominently was in the context of discussing other kinds of chronic illness and author experiences with the medical industrial complex. While Judy, Elizabeth, and Mary all understood that HIV stigma was unique and unlike stigma associated with other kinds of chronic illness, they also saw connections between themselves and other authors with chronic illness. They made these connections primarily through their shared and constant negotiation with medicine, specifically systems of administrative violence.[1] This led all three women to move in and out of their relationship to disability through reading. It is this mobile identification with disability that I seek to explore in this chapter, suggesting that it creates an alternative epistemology for reading illness, one that can be employed in resistance to the diagnostic reading practices explored in part II.

---

1. I borrow this term from critical legal and trans studies scholar Dean Spade.

Diagnostic reading relies on a static and isolated understanding of subjectivity, one where the author is always-already constructed as a singular subject in need of medical intervention. Within the political economy of stigma, author–reader relationships are mediated textually and paratextually through a neoliberal labor market where medical narratives serve as one more product to enhance medical expertise and exacerbate inequality. Specifically, to read diagnostically, one looks for moments of a narrative that correspond to the expectations of that narrative, relying on a narrative predictability central to the circulation of memoir as a product in the neoliberal marketplace. To read diagnostically is to understand authors writing about chronic illness as always in need of medical intervention. This reading practice is a result of the political economy of stigma.

The medical practitioners with whom I have worked all tended to read diagnostically, looking for places where the narrative cohered with their expectations; when this coherence did not exist, the narrative became unpalatable. Even more dangerous than this individual diagnostic reading is the appropriation of narrative by the medical industrial complex, and more specifically, the appropriation of narrative training to create a more skilled and empathetic practitioner. This narrative training turns diagnostic reading into a strategy to be commodified, relying on simplistic understandings of a text to calculate sentence length and diction and categorize medical narratives for the sake of more efficient diagnosis. In the process of this appropriation, those with little access to privacy because of systems of racism, classism, sexism, homophobia, and ableism bear the brunt of administrative violence in the circulation of their stories within medical offices, medical trainings, and even publications. In this chapter, I theorize how medical narratives circulate through a system of administrative violence. I do so by analyzing the disclosures of administrative violence first from accounts with AIDS service workers and then from accounts from my first group of women living with HIV. This analysis provides a scaffold for understanding how reacting to administrative violence leads my research participants living with HIV to develop a reading practice that I call differential reading, in the process resisting diagnostic reading practices inscribed within the political economy of stigma. In adapting Sandoval's idea of differential consciousness to the experience of reading, I am highlighting how reading itself is a complex negotiation of power relations.[2]

---

2. I am not using *differential* in the medical sense of the term, as in a differential diagnosis, the distinguishing between clinical conditions that are similar.

Administrative Power and the
Self-Conscious Mobilization of Identity

It is important to understand power in the lives of women living with HIV not as top-down but as administrative, an understanding that draws from the critical trans work of Dean Spade and reflects on Foucault's analysis of biopower. "Rather than administrative systems merely as responsible for sorting and managing what 'naturally' exists, I argue that administrative systems that classify people actually invent and produce meaning for the categories they administer, and that those categories manage both the population and the distribution of security and vulnerability" (Spade 32). Disability is part of this administrative system, since one files for disability status in order to access resources allocated on the basis of individual rights-based claims (claims that have been made, according to Spade, increasingly difficult for plaintiffs to win). "The twenty-year history of the Americans with Disability Act (ADA) demonstrates disappointing results. Courts have limited the enforcement potential of this law with narrow interpretations of its impact, and people with disabilities remain economically and politically marginalized by systemic ableism" (82). According to Spade, proving discriminatory intent is central and almost impossible in claims made through the ADA, but it also individualizes discrimination into, as critical race theorist Alan Freeman argues, a perpetrator/victim dyad (Spade 84). This is dangerous because this dyad is individualizing (of ableism) and obscures historical context. It also doesn't do anything for redistributing life chances across populations (85–86). Law reform efforts do nothing to alter disciplinary norms (106–9); law reform does nothing to destabilize the political economy of stigma. According to Spade, we have to look at norms that "distribute vulnerability and security" across populations—this includes norms that "establish healthy bodies and minds" (23). "The operation of norms is central to producing the idea of the national body as ever-threatened and to justifying the exclusion of certain populations from programs that distribute life chances (white schools, Social Security benefits, land and housing distribution programs) and the targeting of these same populations for imprisonment and violence" (24). One place where we can see the limits of antidiscrimination law is in the experience with the medical community of women living with HIV. While antidiscrimination laws are in place for medical service for women living with HIV, stigma persists, distributing vulnerability across gender, race, and class for women living with HIV.

Administrative Violence and
Differential Reading Practices

Marge is the one participant in my AIDS service worker reading group who is living with HIV; when she began her work as a patient advocate in October, she had already been participating on the Ryan White Clinic's speakers' bureau for a number of years, talking with medical students and other community members in large and small group settings. As a patient advocate, Marge works with new clients to set up care and help decrease stigma (3/13/2015). Marge, a heterosexual White woman, became infected with HIV after a divorce from her husband; her children were already grown, and Marge was living with her eighty-six-year-old mother at the time of her diagnosis. Marge had been sick for weeks, exhibiting "textbook" signs of HIV infection, including pneumonia and thrush, and kept returning to different area EDs looking for an explanation. Because she was not understood as a being a member of an HIV-risk population, doctors did not test her; when she finally received a diagnosis, "I flipped out. I thought I was going to die. When the doctor came in, he didn't connect me with anybody—the Ryan White center or any social workers. Not like we do now. But one of the nurses on the floor was friends with Diana and told me to talk with her" (5/13/2015). Marge became connected to services because of Diana's activism, not because of any formal protocol. Marge went for a few months without sharing her diagnosis with her family, hiding her paperwork under her bed so her mother would not find out. Eventually, Marge had to come out to her daughter because her HIV physician faxed confidential medical documents to her primary care doctor; her daughter worked in that office and was the first to pull the documents from the fax machine. Marge still has not disclosed her status to her extended family, though she continues to tell her story of living with HIV to the larger public.

I believe that those who signed up to participate in my reading group study did so because they identify personally with the HIV virus and understand themselves as activist-caregivers; I do not believe that this is representative of the larger AIDS service worker community. From what I have witnessed in my own work as a volunteer and as a researcher, there seems to be a division among AIDS service workers: first, there are those like Diana who began this work thirty-five years ago and those like Gretta who witnessed deaths from HIV-related illness early on in the crisis; those like Adam and Nick who identify as part of a larger gay community still disproportionately affected by the crisis; those like Tony who began their work as an intellectual interest and then seek to deepen their understanding through activism and care work; those like Marge who begin their AIDS service work because they themselves become infected; and finally, those who are professionalized social workers who know little of HIV history and have little interest in seeing those living with HIV as a part of their larger community. My anecdotal evidence tells me that the last group is a growing population.

My reading group of AIDS service workers spoke about administrative violence toward people living with HIV in their workplace, emphasizing that though many of them were committed to the struggle for HIV equality, many also just treated their work at the local Ryan White Clinic as any other job. Diana, who has been an AIDS activist since the beginning of the movement, tells the group about her difficulty in getting new co-workers to learn about the movement: "You know, I always give them tapes like 'How to Survive a Plague' and 'We Were There' [two recent HIV documentaries about the early days of the crisis in the US] about the early days of the struggle with HIV and the struggle to get these meds. And let me put it this way: I gave it to people who didn't know a thing about HIV, and it was still on their desk and they never took it home" (6/8/2015). As Gretta recounts in our first full group meeting, "I think there are people in our office, there are people who don't have a passion for HIV and you can tell the difference—they are good at what they do but you can tell they are waiting for the next thing" (5/11/2015). For Gretta this causes more work because there is a lack of interest in their clients and in the larger political project of HIV equality and service. Nick, from his experience in social work classes, believes part of the reason for this lack of passion is that the process of getting a social work degree is too regimented; students do not get to choose classes out of interest but are instead put on a strict track to graduation. This critique resonates with Marge and frustrates her; she is the only member of the group living with HIV (5/11/2015).

In our second meeting, the group shares another strand of what makes their jobs difficult—the lack of knowledge and services in local EDs. HIV screenings are not a part of the regular STD panels or the rape kits. When asked why this is not standard protocol, Diana tells the group: "I hate to put this on tape, but it is standard. It is on the panel of things you check off on the electronic medical records, the doctors ding it, they just won't do it. Because it's either extra work—we went to a conference to talk about why people don't want to test and it's extra work. It's uncomfortable for people" (6/8/2015). Marge echoes this, contributing knowledge from her experience in an administrative capacity for a local family physician. As Diana recounts, HIV service workers and activists have been fighting for EDs to make HIV tests standard protocol for years, with little to no result. On the few occasions when ED doctors and primary care doctors do conduct HIV tests, they contribute little to follow-up care, as Marge's experience attests.

This administrative violence happens also in the context of routine staff conversations in and around the office of the clinic. As Gretta recounts, "We also had a co-worker who, they were new, and they found out we had pregnant patients and she was appalled. And she was talking to me about it in the office and a consumer advocate at the time was sitting outside the door and she came in and was like, 'I have two children'—at the time, now she just had a third—'and I'm positive and my husband is not, and neither are my kids' and this just stopped it. This person was a nurse for many years" (6/8/2015). This violence takes the form of a casual conversation with co-workers, one that can easily be overheard by clients and other co-workers.

Marge and Gretta also share their experience at a recent AIDS service worker conference in Pennsylvania, to learn about client retention, where the dominant conversation was focused around promoting abstinence for those living with HIV. As Gretta tells the group, "I learned more from reading this [holds up Marvelyn Brown's *The Naked Truth: Young, Beautiful, and (HIV) Positive,* our book for the week] on the car ride down" (6/8/2015). As my group members demonstrate, administrative violence functions as stigma turned localized "common sense" within the industry, leading to poor and, as Diana tells it, "unrealistic" policy decisions within ASOs.

Nick also demonstrates how administrative violence works at the level of fundraising. In discussing a recent grant, Nick tells the group a story I have heard many times as a volunteer with several ASOs. "We can only pay for things that are HIV-related. Like if we send somebody to go see a specialist because it is HIV-related or their insurance won't cover something else they need. There is only so much we can provide them financially or whatever for the rest of their health; I mean, we are trying to get a primary care physician for our patients who are less fortunate and do not have one and the grant won't cover it. Everything is HIV-related for these people!" (6/08/2015). For Nick the line between health care and social services that are HIV-related for those living with HIV is an arbitrary one, yet most grant funding works to maintain this rigid line. In our next meeting, the group also discusses how unfortunate it is that the Ryan White Act, our nation's primary financial funding for providing medications and medical services for those living with HIV, itself must be renewed each year by Congress (8/11/2015). I would add that the escalating cost of HIV medications themselves (thousands of dollars a month) is a primary example of administrative violence for the profit of a few.

It is in this context of administrative violence within the medical industrial complex that client narratives circulate. That said, I do believe that life narrative is an important tool for transforming systems of injustice; the Boston Women's Health Collective exemplified some of this importance by the groundbreaking inclusion of personal narratives in their first edition (and all subsequent editions) of *Our Bodies, Ourselves*.[3] Similarly, the disability rights movement also used life narrative to effectively argue for policy change and the passing of the ADA.[4] While we can certainly argue about the various successes of these movements, it is difficult to argue that reading, listening to, and writing life narrative cannot be empowering in a personal and political terrain. But unlike medical practitioners who call for a diagnostic reading practice in order to simplify narratives to fit a for-profit medical model of care, the women I worked with in my first reading group, all of whom were living with HIV and reading memoirs about HIV and other chronic illness, demonstrated a reading practice that I call differential reading. It is this practice that I would like to highlight as an alternative epistemology (cripistemology) for the production, circulation, and reception of life narratives about illness.

I conceptualize my understanding of differential reading from Chicana critical theorist Chela Sandoval and her work on differential consciousness. For Sandoval, differential consciousness is a mobile identification (44). Sandoval understands third-world feminism as providing that theoretical and methodological approach for oppositional consciousness (45–54). The differential is performative in that it relies on a form of agency that is self-consciously mobilizing modes of opposition (57). "The differential mode of social movement and consciousness depends on the practitioners' ability to read the current situation of power and self-consciously choosing or adopting the ideological stand best suited to push against its configurations, a survival skill well-known to oppressed peoples" (59). Sandoval's work on differential consciousness resonates with crip theory, a concept elicited by Robert McRuer and Carrie Sandahl that, in theorist Alison Kafer's summary, "is more contestatory than disability studies, more willing to explore the potential risks and exclusions of identity politics" (2013, 15). As Kafer argues, crip theory is an expansive

---

3. For a full discussion of the women's health movement, see Kathy Davis, *The Making of "Our Bodies, Ourselves": How Feminism Travels Across Borders* (Duke UP, 2007); Wendy Kline, *Bodies of Knowledge: Sexuality, Reproduction, and Women's Health in the Second Wave* (U of Chicago P, 2009); and Sandra Morgen, *Into Our Own Hands: The Women's Health Movement in the United States, 1969–1990* (Rutgers UP).

4. For a full discussion of the disability rights movement, see Sharon Barnatt and Richard Scotch, *Disability Protests: Contentious Politics 1970–1999* (Gallaudet UP, 2001); James I. Charlton, *Nothing About Us Without Us: Disability Oppression and Empowerment* (Berkeley: U of California P, 1998); and Kim E. Nielsen.

theory, including those who both "claim disability identity and desire an end to their own impairments," creating a "paradoxical approach to identity" (16); I would say, in solidarity with Sandoval, a differential approach to identity. The claim of disability relies on one's analysis of power and self-conscious mobilization of resistance to that power. The women in my first reading group demonstrated a self-conscious resistance to medical power by moving in and out of identification with disability; while none of the three women I worked with identified explicitly as disabled, they all identified with other people with disability and used this identification to mobilize a resistance to the medical industry as a whole.

By practicing differential reading, my research participants move in and out of identification with disability itself. Differential reading is both a reading practice for memoirs (between readers and the memoir) and a reading practice that emerges through the collective experience of reading the memoir together. Differential reading generates knowledge systems about disability and illness that resist the top-down reading practice of diagnostic reading so prevalent within the medical industrial complex and in a larger cultural common sense.

Judy: Reading and Resisting through Her Mother's Work

When I first met Judy in the summer of 2012, she was looking for work through a local disability assistance program. Yet, from the beginning of our time together, Judy was adamant that her illness was not a disability: "I'm taking care of myself more now. Drinking water. I started disciplining myself and eating better. Taking a lot of stuff out of my diet. Started adding good stuff, you know, fruit. Lord thank you! He wants me to take care of myself. How can you be any help to Him if you, how can you if you're sick? As far as that, I really don't think of my illness as a disability" (8/23/2012). Here, Judy tells me how her HIV diagnosis has brought her attention to a new regimen of diet and exercise, a regimen encouraged by AIDS service organizations. What is interesting is that this regimen is similar to any advice given about chronic illness: the focus is on curbing individual behavior, often at the high cost of food (Judy lives in an area of the city that might be considered a food desert, with little access to fresh fruit and vegetables, let alone organic, chemical-free produce). Additionally, exercise is difficult because of injuries sustained working in a factory and lack of appropriate clothing, footwear, and inexpensive exercise facilities. What is most interesting to me about Judy's resistance to identifying as disabled here is the twofold insistence that (a) she can do something about her illness (thus, she is not truly disabled), and (b) because of her Christian faith, she must do something or else she is useless to God. In effect, in being able to work to alleviate the symptoms of her illness, she is not truly disabled. Yet, she recognizes not only that disability services are available to her but that she is deserving of these services.

According to Judy, she began applying for disability services because of a deteriorating joint disease, of which the slipped discs in her back were symptomatic. However, she was unable to qualify for disability services while also unable to work; it was not until she received her HIV diagnosis that the combination of her joint disease and her HIV made her an appropriate candidate for disability assistance.[5] Judy also recognizes that in order to be able to be a candidate for a job that "is not too stressful," such as working in an office and answering phones, she needs to learn computer skills, a process she was just beginning when we met in 2012. Still, the goal of having a job was not to completely forgo disability assistance: "I don't want nothing too stressful. And it has to work around my schedule. My church" (August 23, 2012). Thus, disability assistance allows Judy to be in greater service to her church and faith community, a central aspect of her identity.

In one of our early reading group meetings, I learned from Judy that one of her daughters had sickle cell disease, an experience that allowed her and her daughter to become close through countless childhood hospitalizations. When I asked whether she saw any similarities between the experience of her daughter with sickle cell and her own experience with HIV, she replied with an unequivocal "no": "You got the sickle cell disease, it's okay. I got HIV. Oooooooh. You can't say that. There's a difference. Yes it is. I think it's different from anything" (11/1/2012). For Judy the difference between sickle cell and HIV is the personal responsibility that others place on contracting HIV. For Judy, HIV has an origin story that involves sexual transgression and drug abuse, warranting stigma that other chronic illness does not.

While Judy is adamant that HIV is unlike other kinds of chronic illness because of the associated stigma, she is also able to relate the skills she learned advocating for her daughter's care to her own interaction with medical professionals. She also relates her skills, perhaps most poignantly, to her own mother's work as a nurse in the segregated South. In our first reading group meeting, in the process of telling the others in the group about her initial

---

5. It is not my project here to clarify what qualified Judy for disability assistance; what interests me is Judy's understanding of her qualification and how that affects her identity itself.

diagnosis with HIV, Judy also discusses her negotiation of HIV medications. From the beginning when telling the story of her diagnosis, she centralizes her negotiations of medications and her refusal to accept medical treatment that did not agree with her body, since she's allergic to penicillin and sulfur drugs:

> I've been on three regimens because the first one they put me on I started having some problems, I stopped feeling pain within my legs and I was like "Nu-uh. I'm not taking this. And I shouldn't be feeling these cramps in my legs. It's pain. It's unusual pain." I said, "I need a break then." Then they said, "Six months. Then we'll try putting you on something else." They tried me on, 'kay, that wasn't doing what it should. Eventually, they said, "we gonna do this test that kind of tell what different medicines that you would be able to take" [. . .] They said, "ma'am, miss, with your body, a lot of these medicines are not going to agree with you." Ain't nothing new. (10/25/2012)

Judy circles back to her negotiation of medication and doctor visits in our fourth reading group meeting, giving me a chance to ask follow-up questions about how she learned this kind of negotiation strategy:

> It was to a point that they were starting to say it's only medicine we don't have that many selections. I was on this one that was awful. It was—we got so many medicines. You see this? This is the list here that, of the research they've come out with. You are limited. You are limited in this section. And to this section. So now you can't take here and eventually, you're going to be limited, there's only so many that will apply to you. So, I'm like, "Okay, I don't know what to tell you but I'm not going to go on this and that and everything you want to give me either." Then they come out with their test. Uh-huh. I knew something else could be done. (10/25/2012)

I asked Judy when she had learned that she could negotiate with doctors, since many people would never think to talk to their doctors like that if something isn't working. She credited her mother, a nurse, with teaching her how to navigate the medical system:

> She would always tell me, you gotta watch what your doctor, you just can't take, you've got to watch everything the doctor tell you. You gotta get second opinions. Third opinions if you have to. Don't accept anything the doctors tell you. That was one thing right there. Don't accept anything the doctors tell you. Ask the question. Ask questions. (10/25/2012)

What impressed me about Judy from the beginning of our relationship was her assertiveness with her medical team, her recognition of when treatment was not working, and her refusal to accept discomfort and/or pain in treatment:

> Doctors is not, they not always right! Nobody's living in your body but you. You're a doctor. You the nurse. You have the nurse's yourself. You have to walk your walk daily, 24 hours a day, you know how your body feels, you know. If anybody need to be experimenting, I be like, that's my encouraging words, I be like "you experimenting on your own body" might as well. This is a lifetime process. Cause I'm working with the doctors and I'm talking to them and you may have went to school, you might have went to college, but I don't have to go there to know my body, what my body needs every day or how my pain is feeling. You'll never know how my pain is feeling. You only know what I'm telling you. [. . .] I talk to [my doctor] and he's like why don't you try this out. It's cream instead of, um, IB Profen [*sic*] that you been taking. This other stuff. Would you like to try this? And I'm like what are you talking about? I'm going to try you on. Take some home and try what it is. And call me back the next day and see how you like it. I said okay, I'll try it. And he sent it in, no problem. And my pain pills I've been taking. I don't think 1,000 milligrams is really working. It can't be my symptoms. He said well, okay. I also know it's a 1,000 Vicodins [*sic*]—I said, why can't I take 750? And he said, you can. And I said, well great. [laughter] I can try that. I try different things because I want to see what's going on with my situation. I have too much going on with my life not to be, so much going on where I can't do what I need to do, you know, to accomplish my goals and things. (10/25/2012)

Much of my conversation with AIDS service workers revolved around complaints with clients and their (lack of) medication adherence; much of the time this lack of adherence was attributed to either personal addiction or "poor" decision-making or structural barriers. Judy gave me her perspective on taking medication:

> JUDY: I'm going to work with you. You all better work with me because I'm going to work with you. 'Cause I have to do this fight. I'm trying only one pill. I'm still taking them like prescribed. But I'm trying, cutting it [in] half or whatever, I'm going to know. If it makes me too drowsy. 'Cause I've found times when taking too many it just took too many and I'm out. I did a conference at the college, a leadership conference. I volunteered. But I'm sitting in one workshop and I'm passing out information and I take my medicine and I'm sitting there, and I put an extra Vicodin

in there, so I end up taking two plus the IB Profen [*sic*]. I couldn't keep my eyes open. It was so unbelievable awful. And I was like I definitely don't want that! I'm going to be working with them. [. . .]

A: In the class I teach at the university with my students, some of them are really young, like 18, 19, 20, we talk about how to talk to doctors, to encourage them to ask the questions, to ask the follow-up questions; if you don't know what they are prescribing you, ask them what it is.

JUDY: And read the labels! When you do get medicine. Read it all. Fine print. Everything. Read. it. all. They don't want you to read. (10/25/2012)

Never did an AIDS service worker understand that medication adherence could be the result of a complex negotiation of power relations that Judy describes; a reflection of the intersection of physical discomfort/pain and historical generational medical violence written about in relation to African American bodies in particular.[6] That Judy learned this medical negotiation from her mother's work as a nurse is further evidence that recognition of medical power and abuse transcends generations not just through trauma but through creative and astute tactics for resisting this power in the contemporary moment.

This complex negotiation of medical power dynamics that Judy negotiates daily creates the epistemological foundation for her reading about chronic illness. Judy, because of her warranted distrust of medical authority, does not divulge endless intimate details to her medical team; similarly, Judy does not expect the memoirists we read together to provide all intimate details about their lives. In our reading together, Judy consistently finds connections between the experience of memoirists, despite differences in generation, class, race, and illness. One place where I witnessed this kind of reading strategy was our reading of Roxanne Black's *Unexpected Blessings: Stories of Hope and Healing*, a memoir by a young woman with lupus. When I asked Judy what initially struck her in her reading of Black's memoir, she pulled out her book, reading glasses, and read to me a highlighted section of chapter 2: "Love Unconditionally," a passage about how important is can be to connect and bond with others (11/8/2012). Judy elaborates on how important it is to connect with others who experience chronic illness:

When you're sick and you're down, and feeling bad and in pain, it's like who you want to bother with. It's hard. You can, you know, go out with your friends, whoever, and your family, whatever they, you kind of like stray away

---

6. For a more thorough discussion of the abuses of African Americans by the medical field, see Harriet A. Washington, *Medical Apartheid: The Dark History of Medical Experimentation on Black Americans from Colonial Times to Present* (Anchor Books, 2006).

from them, so to speak. Talking to them about it. It depends on how much pain. The pain! It's no joke. You gotta—not all diseases have pain but if you have one that consists of you being in pain, you gotta, you know. Friends might help but because of your attitude, your expressions, you might not be proud of being in pain and hurting. (11/8/2012)

Here, Judy refers to the importance of relationships built around understanding chronic pain specifically. But the emphasis here is not that one could simply understand what another is feeling in a disembodied way but that one can relate to the logistics of managing life around pain. In drawing connections between the experience of lupus and HIV, Judy immediately connects to the necessity of interacting with doctors and the negativity by doctors experienced by Roxanne Black, Catherine Wyatt-Morley, and herself. Judy felt that Wyatt-Morley's doctor "was draining from her spirit." Though she hypothesized that the doctor "didn't want her hopes to get up too high to feel let down," Judy ultimately concludes that to be an effective doctor "you have to be an encouraging person" because "a person who may have an illness that is a death sentence. It could be a death sentence. They need encouragement until their time comes." When asked whether she'd ever experienced that negativity from doctors herself, Judy pauses:

JUDY: Recently. My pain specialist. This new doc. He's a new specialist for me. And he, when I first went to him and stuff and he looked at my records and everything he's like, "You got AIDS. You got AIDS. What in the world? A pretty girl like you doing with AIDS?" He was going like this.

A: Just, like, shaking his head back and forth.

JUDY: Yes. "How did that happen?" So, well, it happened. It just happened. And it was 15 years ago, okay. And the way he said this, he always said "AIDS" as if I was like, we talked about this before, because no, that's not my diagnosis.

A: Shows us how much we need to school physicians. We need to educate physicians. About HIV. In some ways, right?

JUDY: Uh-huh!

A: 'Cause they're not, they're not paying attention to what's happening.

JUDY: It can he hurtful. It really can. If you really don't know about it, and don't know, understand, it's the devil. It's not that person. Saying that stuff.

A: And that's what helps you get through it.

JUDY: Uh-huh. (11/8/2012)

The negativity that memoirist Roxanne Black experiences from her doctors leads Judy to share this story of interacting with her pain specialist. Judy discloses these details to me in the context of finding similarities across illnesses, similarities that reflect her constant attention to medical power. In later meetings, Judy will find similar connections in reading Danquah's *Willow Weep for Me*, linking depression to HIV (1/24/2013, 2/28/2014). In a final link between HIV and other medical conditions, Judy discloses in our final reading group meeting her sister's hysterectomy and her own opportunity to serve as a medical liaison and expert on her sister's behalf. While Judy does not talk with her sister directly about her HIV status very often, her sister turns to Judy for help in negotiating her care with her medical team before and after her hysterectomy, an indicator that Judy's experience negotiating her own medical care is transferrable beyond HIV (3/7/2013).

In my final one-on-one interview with Judy, I asked again about disability identification, since over the course of our time together I saw her making connections with others with chronic illness through her experience negotiating medical care. Judy expressed her feelings of satisfaction with the reading group: "The books helped to encourage me. I was encouraged by the books because they helped me to understand that I also can start writing as well, and that a lot of womens [sic] are out there who do have the boldness to share their experience with HIV. And AIDS. And other illnesses. Any illness" (3/26/2013). Here, Judy connects HIV to other illnesses, particularly through the power of writing and disclosure.

At an earlier meeting, I ask Judy whether she feels like HIV is a part of her identity.

JUDY: I think HIV is disappeared, gone actually! In my life, yah. This is what it is:

A: Okay.

JUDY: My T-cell count is rising every four months. And what seems clear to me is HIV is no longer, I am definitely not living with HIV but HIV may be living with me! (11/8/2012)

Because Judy is satisfied with her HIV care team and her medication regimen, she no longer feels that HIV is a prominent part of her life.

JUDY: I had an appointment last week right for my checkup and I almost forgot actually. 'Cause it wasn't a primary focus. 'Cause I wasn't primary focuses [sic] on okay, I got this appointment. What my T-cell count was

gonna be, how low it was going to be, or I just—I totally almost forgot
until two or three hours before it's time for the appointment!

A: Yah.

JUDY: I'm like, wow, I have an appointment today! Well, I go in and I think
nothing of it. It's like okay, I got an appointment,

A: Yah, it's just like a regular part of your routine.

JUDY: Uh-huh. I'm doing what I supposed to be doing. I'm taking my meds
and things. I take them no matter because the reports says one thing and
that you know, it look unknown but in reality, we go by numbers and
we going by bloodwork from the beginning. I feel like this, I'm healed.
Totally. I feel like God has healed me! My T-cell count was 1,500, it's
1,800 now. That's evidence that a miracle has happened. If I didn't have
evidence that a miracle has happened, that would be something different. But I'm having evidence all of the sudden in my life, I'm having
evidence of a miracle.

Judy's reference to her spirituality and Christian faith echoes the experience and narrative of Wyatt-Morley. In the reading group with AIDS service
workers, Adam set up a bifurcation between memoirists who were "intellectual" and those who were "spiritual," and yet Judy's experience would question
that binary. Judy is both a person with a religious life and someone who thinks
very critically about medical negotiations, structural injustice, and the role
of writing. While Judy has seen her health improve in terms of T-cell counts
(rising) and viral loads (lessening), what is important is that she no longer
experiences the daily labor of managing the power relations with medical doctors. It is these power relations specifically that allow her to make connections
between her HIV experience and other women's experiences with chronic illness. Yet, for Judy, HIV stands apart from other kinds of disability because of
the persistence of stigma:

A: How do you see your experience, um, of, I'm going to use your words,
HIV living with you, as similar or different from living with other kinds
of illness? So we read a couple other books about—we read about a
woman with lupus, a woman with depression, do you think there are
similarities in terms of experience with HIV and those kinds of illnesses
or do you think it's so different that it's hard to make a comparison?

JUDY: Oh, I think it's different. I really do. [pause] Any other illness can be
shared, freely; HIV, on the other hand, can—it is off in another whole
group by itself. Group. [pause] Cancer, cancer cancer. Can be spoke of
so freely these days and times and any other parts of illnesses like dia-

betes—people are quick to say I am a diabetic. Do you think people are going to be quick—and, and this is my opinion—I'm not going to be quick to say I'm HIV like a person would say I'm a diabetic. Or I have lupus.

A: Or sickle cell, like your daughter.

JUDY: Or sickle cell! I have sickle cell, quickly, freely.

A: And is that because of the stigma with HIV?

JUDY: Yah, I think it's because of the stigma. It's because I do not want that stigma. I mean, I'm thinking, I know what they say, you can't get it this way, you can't get it this way, but still! This HIV and AIDS—"I don't want it." Versus anything else. I will definitely as much as possible be staying away from it.

What makes HIV distinct from other kinds of disability for Judy is, first, the stigma associated with HIV origin stories; for Judy, HIV always comes with the expectation that there is an origin story involving sex and drugs.

JUDY: I don't know if people look at it like it's a sexual thing or not—basically, I think it's focused on the sexual versus okay, getting it from a transfusion. You would not even know! Unless they say—you know—because that would probably be the next question: how did you get it?

A: Or who gave it to you.

JUDY: Yes! How did you become infected? How? Because there are so many ways it's like how did you become infected?

What also becomes important for Judy, when I ask directly about disability and being disabled, is her awareness of how the state manages who is allowed to become disabled, who can access benefits.

A: Um. Let me ask you this. So, because HIV is living with you—I really love the way you say that!—because HIV is living with you, um, you have access to some disability resources, are you more or less likely to access those resources after spending time in this reading group? Or not? Are you not really thinking about disability in terms of yourself with a disability?

JUDY: [pause] um. I mean, rephrase that.

Just like Judy narrated to me about her relationships with doctors, she is making me talk to her on her own terms. I complied, mentioning laws that label her as someone with a disability and asking for her thoughts. After noting the paradoxical difficulty of getting the benefits the disability label entitles her to (noted in the last chapter), Judy considered her status in relationship to work and labor.

> JUDY: From what I heard, during my session of disability, I was questioned so hard because I was told, also, you are able to work. Even with it. You are able. You are still able to work. You know?
>
> A: Yah.
>
> JUDY: That's what I was told. You are still abled. They don't look at what's working on the inside. It's what's working on the outside, too, you know? You all your body parts are working, there is something you can do. There is something a person can do. Just sitting, passing out something. It's something they can do. What you gotta be dying to get it? On your deathbed? Now AIDS on the other hand, that might make a difference. When it comes down to being disabled. But HIV alone? My understanding is that you are not going to be considered disabled.

For Judy, disability is not a consciousness that is unmediated by the state, yet Judy's precise understanding of how disability identity works, and her willingness to engage with disability identification in order to access resources, highlights her differential negotiation of identity. Further, Judy's ability to find connections with others experiencing disability or chronic illness through their shared negotiation of medical services highlights how life writing can be used to subvert the political economy of stigma and medical power.

Elizabeth: Reading across Differences to Make Change

As I discussed in my first chapter, when I first met Elizabeth, she understood HIV as a part of her identity, primarily because it was something she had to think about and manage daily. This experience of the daily management of chronic illness did not fade for Elizabeth during our time together. In our final interview, I asked her about similarities between living with HIV and living with other kinds of chronic illness or disability. She responded by describing how "living with a diagnosis" of any kind changes one's "mindset" and prompts not only a "lifestyle change" but also "a self-image change":

> You're not as—what's the word I want to use?—careless. You're more conscious of your decisions and choices you make. Especially when it comes to relationships. Um. How you want to be treated. And how you really want,

you know, to, I think, better yourself. I think, for me, that's for me it's how do I want to better my life? You know. (3/13/2013)

In this discussion, Elizabeth helped me understand that the connection she makes between living with HIV and living with other chronic illnesses is one of daily management—changing one's lifestyle and navigating medical decisions, certainly, but also about how the vulnerability of a chronic illness diagnosis allows her the opportunity to "set boundaries" in her relationships with others. Before her diagnosis, Elizabeth said, "I didn't have no self-confidence," but since then, "I've really started to look inside myself, you know, what do I want, what am I going to put up with." At the same time, Elizabeth also draws a clear distinction between understanding herself as a part of the disability community; for her, the label of disability works like a firm boundary between herself and work.

> ELIZABETH: I don't want to lessen the, you know, the fact that I do have HIV, but I don't want it to be a barrier. So, I don't want to look at myself as disabled. That's why I've got this "I've gotta get off disability, I gotta go back to work, to do something to feel like I am a part of society. Instead of taking from society." You know what I mean? Giving back more.
>
> A: So, if you don't see yourself as a woman with a disability, and you totally explained that really well, do you see yourself as working with a group of women, coming together working with or having a support group with other women who have chronic illness or disability? Do you see yourself as part of that bigger picture?
>
> ELIZABETH: Yes, I do, most definitely. In the beginning I didn't think it was going to be possible but after reading these books and doing a lot of self-discovery.

In discussing the memoirs that we read together, Elizabeth is indeed inspired; but for Elizabeth, she is not inspired as an able-bodied person by a disabled person but as a chronically ill person inspired to create a different kind of life for herself by witnessing another chronically ill person also make significant changes. Elizabeth frequently talks about herself as a "helper" and "caregiver" and not someone who is "like poor me, poor me"—helping me to understand that her inspiration is to work in the community.

Ironically, Elizabeth, who lives with the effects of a stroke and cannot use her left hand for typing or writing, expresses her desire early on to write about her experiences with HIV but is unable to do so until she discovers voice recognition software (1/17/2013). Elizabeth relays this information (about the stroke and her limited mobility, which is not apparent to me even after several meetings with each other) only in the context of reading about other disability and accommodations. The experience of managing illness or disability in the context of the memoirs is what leads to Elizabeth's disclosure; like Judy, I believe this is also an important epistemology for accessing these memoirs. Elizabeth makes connections between her experiences with disability and illness when she reads about, and the group discusses, their management of various medical conditions and diagnosis. Their relationship to the labor of navigating medical systems leads to their differential reading strategies.

While the daily management of illness leads to a differential reading strategy, the stigma related to HIV specifically leads all the group participants to continue to understand HIV as a distinct experience that disallows intimacy with other people with chronic illness. Elizabeth explains her experience with stigma this way:

> Heavyset people, overweight people they are ostracized, they are talked about, you know, to a certain extent, you know? But you let someone say, well I have HIV, oh my god, the world would fall, you know, if sometimes it feels like if you just, if the world is just crumbling around you and you are on this pedestal and everyone is just looking up at you like, all eyes on me, you know, type deal [. . .] And all of the sudden, you are in a crowd, and everything else just falls down to the side. And everyone is just looking up at ya. (2/07/2013)

Here, by relating to others with chronic illness (such as heart problems or depression), Elizabeth is able to formulate how HIV is so different. Elizabeth talks with me a few times about her heart problems, which some might not expect because she does not fit the stereotype of obese or overweight. Elizabeth recognizes that she is not stigmatized because of how she looks despite having a heart condition that many overweight people are stigmatized for having (whether or not they do). She also connects HIV to her own depression, another invisible condition whose symptoms (low energy, sadness) others misread as laziness, particularly when embodied by a Black woman. While Elizabeth is able to make connections between HIV and two other invisible chronic illnesses she experiences, she is also adamant that HIV is different. She reiterates what resonates with all my group participants—that HIV stigma is closely connected to assumptions about origin stories. Although HIV stigma does cause Elizabeth to feel isolated from others, she also recognizes how these feelings of isolation connect to the depression that Danquah writes about in *Willow Weep for Me*:

With that one, with *Willow Weep for Me,* because I know I have dealt with depression for a long time. Um, and then, not knowing what it was that was going on with me. And then reading her story, I was like, "That's what it was! Okay, now I know," but the depression is more, I think, the difference between the depression and the HIV; I think the difference is a lot of people get depressed. More so than you know the majority that doesn't, you know, but in the same sense with both situations, you are not willing to admit it, to look into it—you are willing to ignore it instead of really delving into and being like what is going on with me and really find out. You know, it will go away. Or I'll just hide away, and it will go away, type deal. And in both situations, you're going through the same thing. I'll hide and nobody will know. I'll isolate and nobody will know. But in the same sense, they both eat away at the soul of you, and the core of who you are and who you can be. (2/7/2013)

Through her technique of differential reading, Elizabeth is able to clearly articulate similarities to and differences from HIV, theorizing from her own experience without disclosing unnecessary personal details. Elizabeth is not offering me, her listener, details of her life story so much as she is making organic comparisons and associations that help us both understand the experience of HIV more viscerally and clearly. The books themselves are conduits allowing us to maintain boundaries with one another in order to focus on the ideas of the text itself.

By the end of our time together, Elizabeth reflects on the experience of reading together. I asked her in our final one-on-one interview what she thought about reading together, particularly given that in our first interview, she didn't identify herself as a reader. During that interview, she mentioned that she was interested in reading more, but that may have just been because I was recruiting for a reading group; she may have just been willing to go to any group of women living with HIV, regardless of the activity, since there was none available in town at the time. In our meetings together, there was never any pressure to read at a certain pace or even to complete the books we chose. All participants received free books and could do whatever they pleased with them. My question for Elizabeth about her perspective on reading was one of open curiosity, with no expectation of a particular answer:

I liked it. First and foremost, because it was so informatable [*sic*]. I've gotten so much information for myself about my health, about my diagnosis, I've learned a few things I didn't even know that brought, you know, brought to

light for me and I'm so appreciative for it. I really enjoyed it. I really did.
Especially getting into, getting back into reading. Getting into the books, you
know? And that was really nice. I liked it. (3/13/2013)

While access to the books themselves was helpful for Elizabeth, I believe the
process of differential reading requires conversations with peers. Through
finding commonalities with and differences from one another's personal
experiences and their readings of the memoirs, my first group participants,
all women living with HIV, were able to more effectively use their reading of
memoirs. By *effectively*, I mean that reading—for Elizabeth and other members of the first reading group—led to recognition and change, a key effect of
differential reading.

Elizabeth confirmed my suspicions. When I asked whether she learned
more from the books or from other group members, she enthusiastically
replied, "Both!" When asked whether she was likely to read more autobiography going forward, she responded with an equally enthusiastic "Oh yes!"

Especially with the subject matter that we've been dealing with. You know,
the diagnosis of the HIV. And the mental health diagnosis. I think it helps
to find out how others worked their way through a lot of things, you know,
obstacles; it brought to light a lot of things I needed to check out for myself.
I think I'll always [*sic*], I love autobiographies now. [laughing] (3/13/2013)

All women found themselves making changes in their own lives in the process
of our meeting together; for Elizabeth these changes were directly connected
to reading memoir.

Mary: Resisting through Relationships

Mary was the research participant in my first group who came to the fewest
group meetings and read the least amount of material; as a result, I had difficulty getting to know her and her reading strategies, although she was always
forthcoming about her personal experiences with HIV illness. She and I were
both White women of about the same age, and, as a result, she often related
to me as a peer as we swapped stories about early childhood fascinations with
Paula Abdul and *Saved by the Bell* and of high school in the 1990s.

When I met Mary in October 2012, she had been living with HIV for four
years, had been involved with the local AIDS service organization for three,

and had never found a group specifically for women living with HIV. Not having a group for women in town was a significant oversight because of the stigma that heterosexual women feel and experience when trying to date while living with HIV (10/22/2012). When I ask Mary in our first meeting whether she understands herself as a part of a disability community, she is adamant that she is not disabled. She does mention in this meeting that she is in the middle of a workers' compensation lawsuit that is workplace-related; when I ask follow-up questions about the Americans with Disability Act, she is unaware of this legislation. During this meeting, she also mentions that she has never read a full book before and is not particularly looking forward to reading memoir.

As our time went on in our reading group together, Mary was very attentive to listening to the memoir synopsis, asking other group members follow-up questions about the books, and finding connections with her own experiences. One aspect of Mary's experience that she does recount a few times is the process of diagnosis, which for Mary involved months of blood work and misdiagnosis. She was initially diagnosed with lymphoma (10/12/2012). Mary's experience with misdiagnosis and the months of physical illness and depression that followed her initial exposure give her plenty of places to share her personal experience and connections with both our memoirists and other group members.

It is in the process of sharing their experiences of negotiating with medical personnel that we learn that Mary is in a different position from other members of the group; despite her being seropositive for four years, Mary's viral load remains undetectable, a rare condition that allows her to delay a pharmaceutical regimen for up to fifteen years. This reveal prompts the participants to compare notes about their journeys in medical care.

ELIZABETH: By the praise of God, I've only had to try one medication and no side effects whatsoever. I've been blessed in that area.
MARY: Just one pill?
ELIZABETH: Just one pill.
MARY: That's awesome.
ELIZABETH: Yes.
MARY: See? That's my scary. I'm scared when I hit that it will be reality.
ELIZABETH: Actually, it's three.
JUDY: In one. You do the three in one?
ELIZABETH: Yes.
JUDY: I got three. I take three. One of them I know has got two or three different medications.

[pause]

ELIZABETH: And this is like the time I seen. When I first got my medication, my doctor told me I'll see you back in six months. And then I went

MARY: [interrupting] When you first started it?

ELIZABETH: Yah.

MARY: When your counts are that low? My gosh!

ELIZABETH: I had been in and out of the hospital

MARY: I would think two weeks

ELIZABETH: All last year

MARY: Why were you sick?

ELIZABETH: Just pneumonia.

MARY: So, the acute stage? OR is this while you were on meds?

ELIZABETH: No, this is before I had even started meds.

MARY: Oh, okay. They didn't give you a vaccine immediately? I don't even. I
took so many shots when I was diagnosed!

ELIZABETH: [muffled]

MARY: The first thing they said to me was get your pneumonia vaccine

A: Everybody has different, kind of, treatment.

[Lots of talking over each other excitedly]

ELIZABETH: Your metabolism

JUDY: The whole makeup is different

ELIZABETH: Right

MARY: Plus, I have my mom as a doctor over here like "give her everything"

ELIZABETH: I didn't find out about that [the vaccine] until visiting [the local
children's museum].

[group laughter, chatting about the human body exhibit] (10/12/2012)

The negotiation of medical care consistently inspired this kind of fast, excited
conversation among my group participants. Here, Mary asks both Elizabeth
and Judy about their experience on medication since she is not yet taking any
HIV meds; when she finds out that Elizabeth's doctor prescribed her medications for the first time with a six-month follow-up appointment, as opposed
to an appointment in a couple of weeks, and did not recommend a pneumonia
vaccine, she is surprised at Elizabeth's doctor's lack of care. The group breaks
the seriousness of this conversation when Elizabeth admits her own lack of
knowledge about vaccines through referring to the local children's museum's
current exhibit as her key site of education. Whether this is true or not for
Elizabeth, the reference to the local children's museum builds camaraderie
among the group during our first meeting together.

In our final interview together, I ask Mary about her experience with the reading group. While she admits that she read very little of the memoirs along the way because of a lack of time, she did find her time with the group of women living with HIV to be invaluable. She continued to ask the AIDS service organization about hosting a support group for women with HIV. As Mary tells me, "I just don't think they have enough interested. What they say is women—what were they telling me? She explained it as the women who do have it have children and is more focused on their family than they are in really opening up and looking to have camaraderie with their disease. Versus me being single and having no kids—there aren't many people in my situation" (4/1/2013). The explanation Mary was given by the ASO staff speaks to the sexism of the establishment that increases the feelings of isolation among the women I worked with who are living with HIV.

I also ask Mary whether she feels HIV is a significant part of her identity. For both Elizabeth and Judy, HIV was a part of their identity, though Judy, in our final interview, reversed the power of living with HIV by saying "HIV is living with me," a gesture toward understanding herself as being in control of her health. For Mary, my question about HIV identity is about whether she is "feeling it." In answering my question about HIV, she goes back and forth in trying to figure out how big of a part of her life it is.

MARY: [pause] You know, in the beginning, it was so much a part of me I wanted to do everything, included, you know, every news TV, every walk, I was so intrigued. And wanted to work within the industry and try, try, try. And just got—didn't get anywhere. So, and you know, my life in the past six months. So honestly, it doesn't cross my mind. I don't know how to make it—I know that doesn't sound right. I haven't been dating so I don't think about it because the only reason I'd be talking about it is if I'm dating and I'm interested in someone. And, you know, before I was very you know, this guy, this guy, this guy. And I'd tell them all and they would care, didn't care, and now I just, I really don't want to meet anybody new. I'm just not in that mood right now. I'm just more my life is turned upside down and I have problems here, and problems there and the HIV actually is just kind of in the background, just because of life itself. Which is good—well, I wish that was the only thing I had to worry about. Because in the beginning, I just wanted to know everything. And do everything. And now I'm just kind of like "eh." God will take care of me. So, it's in the back of my mind. Instead of at the forefront. I mean, I saw friends from 15 years ago and you know, we were conversating and it was kind of like do I tell them? do I not? And I didn't, it was just kind of like, "I wonder if they know." There was, as I said, that commercial. Some friends saw it and people put stuff on Facebook and called my sister so I think those people had an idea but they didn't bring it up and there was nothing but . . . I really don't talk about it much. Unless I'm having a back procedure and they ask, you know, what are your problems?

A: Right. Unless it's more medical.

MARY: Right. Of course, I pray about it. But I don't really have it at the forefront like it was for a long time.

A: If you, if HIV is not part of your identity—

MARY: I mean, it is when it comes to relationships! I mean, it's part of me, like my hair is brown but—I just don't—I don't know. (4/1/2013)

For Mary, her commitment to disclosure in "relationships" applies not only to sexual partners but also to platonic friendships and even interactions with her pedicurist.

MARY: So, I needed a pedicure. Get my feet soaked. And my nail guy knows I have HIV—

A: Yah, you mentioned him before.

MARY: He was funny with me. So today, with the pedicure, he had his gloves on and he was using an instrument to do it and he saw the crack and he goes, "Ew!" and he stopped. He didn't—he stopped that area and did whatever else he was doing. I was like, give me that! I just took the thing from him and I took it off because he wasn't going to do it. It freaked him out. And I know that's what he was thinking. But I didn't say, you're an asshole. I didn't question him. I just said give it to me. 'Cause I'm paying for a pedicure, so I'm getting—so my heel is smooth now, but you know, that scared him. But, I don't know. I just—everything else is so heavy on me right now I just went right over it. Even though that hit me for a quick second. Screw you. I just [laughing] just kind of how it is. So, it's situations like that where the situation goes, "oh shit I have HIV" but I just—I don't know. I fear for the future. But then I see the future being okay. But then some other people not. Ehhhh—I don't know. (4/1/2013)

How much Mary has to negotiate care and disclose HIV is what affects how important HIV is in her life. She mentions that since she has had other "bad" things happening in her life that HIV has taken a back seat; what is interesting to me is that a huge part of these recent negative experiences, particularly her unsuccessful workers' compensation case, are directly related to HIV. Despite her going back and forth about whether HIV is a part of her identity or not, she is still clear that she does not identify as disabled and would not access disability resources. Despite this, when I ask Mary whether she could see herself joining a group with other women with illness or disability, she tells me that she has already joined a group like this in her church, something she did not see herself doing before joining our reading group.

Differential Reading as a Bioethical Future

The reading strategies of the women living with HIV in my first reading group—strategies that involved triangulating personal experience negotiating the medical industrial complex, relating and asking questions of one another, and relating to the memoirists through medical labor—led to a kind of differential consciousness, a kind of consciousness theorized first by Chicana feminist theorist Chela Sandoval. This reading strategy, which I call differential reading, works in opposition to the diagnostic reading of medical practitioners that I explored in part II. Here, readers theorize knowledge through medical negotiations and in coalition with others having similar conditions, understanding this knowledge as necessarily incomplete. This differential reading leads to a differential negotiation of disability identity, a mobile identification where my group members living with HIV both resisted and found coalition with other disability-identified people. Significantly, labor remained central to their identifications; negotiating the labor of their own medical care allowed them to identify with other disabled people, whereas their assumptions about being able to work in the future, to have paid careers, led them to resist a disability identification. The stigma that all three of the group members believed made HIV distinct from other kinds of disability is a stigma mediated and circulated through practices of diagnostic reading.

I want to propose that the differential reading strategy these reading group participants demonstrated can serve as a bioethical model for transforming our relationship to disability memoir as medical practitioners and disability activists alike. Feminist bioethicist Jackie Scully calls for bioethical research to "elicit the idiographic, phenomenological accounts of disabled people" (49). We also need to look at the "patterns and procedures" that marginalize the experiences and opinions of disabled people (49). Differential reading can do just this; however, unlike a medical practitioner reading the experience of a single disabled person through a diagnostic practice, differential reading develops in coalition with other disabled people, drawing knowledge through similarities and differences, contradictions and alliances.

As Scully reminds us, it is difficult for anyone without an impairment to accurately imagine life with impairment; bioethics traditionally tries to overcome this through an exercise of moral imagination (52). Questioning both bioethics and feminist philosopher Maria Lugones, Scully proposes that there are several challenges to moral imagination: first, we imagine another's experience but as ourselves, meaning that we may not be able to walk but that everything about our character remains the same; second, even if we put ourselves in the other's shoes, there are still so many aspects we can't know about that we end up with a mixture of ourselves in the projection (54–56). For Scully, imagination itself is fundamentally embodied (55). Differential reading places embodiment as central to the construction of knowledge; we see this centrality of embodiment in the consistent negotiation of medical care by readers and memoirists. In fact, chronic illnesses in particular demand a centralization of negotiating medical care because the daily condition of the body itself is mobile. The need for medications and other medical interventions cannot be ignored when contracting pneumonia; for someone with an impaired immune system it can lead to death.

A practice of differential reading happens in the relationship between the reader(s) with similar experiences and the memoirists, hinged on the negotiation of the medical industrial complex. None of these relationships are static; they require a constant attention to the mobility of identity and bodies. This practice can undermine diagnostic reading and provide resistance to the political economy of stigma. The boundaries between the experience of the reader(s) and the author, in this differential formulation of knowledge, are also mobile. As Margrit Shildrick contends, if bodies are not fixed, then neither are ethical relationships (11). Shildrick argues that the body, as we understand it, is an inconsistent artifact with many discourses competing at once; some discourses achieve dominance through normalization (13). Through differential reading, no single discourse can achieve dominance. Here, too, normalization is at once recognized and resisted.

Scully argues that it is precisely embodied difference that can lead to different moral understandings. In bridging arguments in disability studies and bioethics, Scully begins with an understanding that one's embodied experience shapes one's moral understanding (8–16). Scully distinguishes between the ethics of disability, which she argues is a "systematic reflection of the morally correct ways to behave toward disabled people," and a disability ethics, which is "particular moral understandings that are generated through the experience of impairments" (9). Scully is mostly concerned with the latter. One reason for the schism between bioethics and disability studies is that bioethics takes a normative approach, "justifying regulatory frameworks established in biomedicine and biotechnology" (10). As Shildrick writes, "Modern biomedicine, whether concerned with the single patient or with populations, is characterized by the strategies of normalization which constantly measure, assess, record, and project the limits of health. But far from being the 'sick' body, which is the center of such surveillance, it is increasingly the case that the body in what is classed as good health must also submit to monitoring" (57). Practices such as diagnostic reading are consistently concerned with processes of normalization at the expense of privacy; differential reading resists biomedical measurement in the production of knowledge.

In his call for interventions in the future of bioethics, bioethicist Howard Brody asks for more dialogue between people at the grassroots level and between disciplines in developing medical care (21–40, 90–100). In drawing on the work of Anne Hudson Jones, he distinguishes between narrative bioethics and narrative approaches to bioethics: narrative bioethics reconceptualizes the basic methods of bioethics. Brody writes, "As narratives are the basic building blocks of moral thought, one can refute or correct a flawed or incomplete narrative only with a better narrative. The interplay between narratives and counternarratives is therefore a critical process of narrative bioethics" (24). While I agree with Brody that we need to understand narratives themselves in communication with one another, I disagree that narratives "replace" one another, particularly if they are "incomplete" or "flawed." In fact, it is precisely because narratives are incomplete and flawed that they are so useful; differential reading strategies provide one way to access this utility and resist the political economy of stigma.

CONCLUSION

Disability, Debility, and Reading for Unruly Subjectivity

This has been a funny project to write. This, in some ways, is a book about books and about whose story matters enough to warrant a publisher's interest, a medical practitioner's understanding, a policymaker's interventions, or an academic's theorizing. We may also think of this book as being about the production of debility, what Jasbir Puar describes as the assemblage of mechanisms at work that "recognizes some disabilities at the expense of other disabilities that do not fit the respectability and empowerment models of disability progress" (xvii). Puar's theory works to outline precisely how disability and ability operate; how some bodies are already understood as ready to be maimed, as debilitated. Debility works to foreclose access to resources and legibility as a disabled subject (ix–31). This project about storytelling is a project about legibility and about who is legible as a disabled subject.

To explore this question of legibility and disability, a question spurred by the work of Joan Scott and of Gayatri Spivak (a genesis shared by Puar when she returns to this seminal text in her prefix to *The Right to Maim*), I began with my own reading of contemporary American women's HIV narratives and the salient connections and disconnections to other disability memoir frequently critiqued within disability studies. I wondered why the cadre of HIV life writing by women has not been theorized through disability studies and what new ways to understand life writing, citizenship, and stigma these authors provided their readers. To think through these relationships between texts and their readers, I began to think about how disability life writing itself circulates within a political economy of stigma, reinforcing our ideas about belonging and citizenship along an intersectional axis of oppression. Ellen Samuels, building on Benedict Anderson's understanding that national coherence emerges through a forgetting of historical violence and incoherence, argues that fantasies of identification—narratives about belonging that emerge in the mid-nineteenth century and circulate through biocertification in the twenty-first century—"are driven by a desire for incontrovertible physical identification so intense that it produces its own realization at the same time that it reinterprets that realization as natural and inevitable" (3). In examining the dialectic between "text, body and nation," Samuels astutely argues that these narratives are concerned not so much with the individual but with "placing that individual within a legible group" (6). In the twenty-first century, bureaucratic documents "purporting to authenticate a person's biological membership in a regulated group" (9), what Samuels calls biocertification, have proliferated, from medicolegal practices of DNA testing to blood quantum legislation. Life narratives emerge in tandem and in tension with these practices of biocertification, which, as Samuels theorizes, rely on "the authority of the expert whose authoritative gaze trumps not only the individual's appearance but, more disturbingly, their own narrative of bodily and social identity" (17). My project, then, of looking at HIV life narratives—both those published and those collected through my reading group research—is to question how these fantasies of identification play out in relation to other bureaucratic systems (HIV blood-testing practices, welfare claims, SSI claims). Life narratives are shaped by practices of biocertification—both in affirmation of and in resistance to these practices. My research reveals, however, that these narratives are not predetermined by the creator but interpreted with each new circulation, interpreted within the political economy of stigma.

In order to deepen my understanding of both HIV life writing and disability life writing more broadly, I conducted reading groups in two rust-belt cities—one with women living with HIV and one with AIDS service workers. To my knowledge, even with the often-theorized disability life-writing memoirs, nothing has been written about how groups of readers respond to these texts, particularly when those readers are disabled and/or marginalized by ableism and the medical industrial complex themselves. These rust-belt reading groups served as both a way to theorize within a community of those directly affected by HIV about HIV life writing and a way to record experiences of my participants, the life-writing working here as a conduit for multiple and contradictory disclosures. What I found in my research was a stark contrast in reader interactions with life writing, leading me to consider the larger field of the medical humanities, and the brand of narrative medicine in particular, and this idea that more disclosure will simply lead to greater empathy and better treatment models and interventions. Rebecca Garden perhaps most importantly traced the problem in the medical humanities with this notion of empathy, an approach that is touted for increasing "patient compliance with therapeutic regimens and increased therapeutic well-being" (2007, 552). As Garden writes, "The problem with empathy begins with a preoccupation with the self that obscures the other. Empathy depends on the experiences and imagination of the person who is empathizing, and this dependency has the potential to obfuscate or exclude the patient's suffering or the meaning the patient makes of suffering" (555). As Garden reminds us, empathy does nothing to change the power relationships within medicine; how clinical empathy is taught does very little to actually address social inequities imbedded in health care itself. My work has shown precisely the dangerous mechanisms in operation within one particular medical humanities practice, narrative medicine; not only does this practice do little to address social inequality; it actually obscures or distorts the social inequalities that undergird diverse medical conditions like the experience of living with HIV.

Within a neoliberal context where the solution to individual illness is individual responsibility, empathy becomes another means by which medical compliance overrides personal well-being. In this formulation, one is deserving of empathy when one is able to comply with medical parameters of care. In other words, resisting stigma in relation to a medical condition depends on one's own medical labor to address that condition.

The political economy of stigma has never been more robust, and this emphasis on patient compliance is central. Compliance is individual patient labor focused on the self, not on addressing larger social and structural inequalities. As Catherine Gouge explains:

> The Compliance 1.0 paradigm assumes that patients are autonomous subjects making choices and taking an "active role" in their own care (though what can count as active is defined by others), and noncompliance, defined in opposition to this, is considered to be passive and self-destructive, a failure to make the right choices about care and cope with treatment. Those who are not compliant are thought to be interfering with treatment, as best, and posing dangerous (even malicious) public health threats at worst. (119)

The emphasis on compliance by contemporary health-care providers and structures falls in line with new innovations in the Ryan White Care Act, traced in detail by medical sociologist Alyson O'Daniel. O'Daniel writes of the experience of African American women with HIV with attention to the material conditions of poverty as "shaped by global neoliberalism" (1–3). Within this spread of neoliberal governance, "the role of the state is to provide for citizens via the maintenance of free-market capitalism"; within this model, poverty itself is the failure of one to adapt to the demands of the free market (3–4). When it comes to HIV/AIDS funding, however, the neoliberal economy is not without its contradictions. "While neoliberal governance may be partially characterized by the divestment of state-sponsored antipoverty programs, it has also ushered in an era of *increased* interest in public funding for HIV/AIDS prevention and care (Susser 2009). The result has been a global scale-up of HIV/AIDS care organized around the understanding that the global HIV/AIDS pandemic is a development problem that threatens international security, free market capitalism (O'Manique 2004), and, ultimately, Western imperialism" (Susser 2009, 5). In her decade-long research study of women living with HIV in the American South, O'Daniel found that because of policy changes, many times women's health and daily life stability were "thwarted" (6). In O'Daniel's analysis, much of this is related to how the Ryan White Care Act "has become entangled in questions of social belonging and historically given dynamics of racism and gender inequality," particularly as they relate to beliefs about personal responsibility (20–25). Congress scaled up HIV/AIDS programming just as it scaled down public antipoverty programs (35). In 2006 the Ryan White Act was up for reauthorization again; African Americans represented 73 percent of new cases (38–40). The reauthorization of the act, known as the Treatment Modernization Act, restricted antipoverty provisions, cutting funding for things like emergency financial assistance, transportation assistance, and case management. In addition, in order to receive any services under Ryan White, those living with HIV have to submit proof of regular medical care in the form of CD4 cell count laboratory tests (42–45). This new rendition of HIV care is strictly about medical service and medical outcome (44–45). This medicalization is accompanied by the "professionalizing" of AIDS service organizations, which includes a preference for employees to have specialized credentials and the phasing out or complete exclusion of peer counseling (51–53). This all reinforces what Watkins-Hayes calls the test-and-treat revolution (178–203). O'Daniel finds in her research that AIDS service workers too often understand the population with whom they work as homogenous with "uniform healthcare needs" (75). Clients were understood as "aggressive" and "engaged in self-defeating strategies"; "employees gave the impression that they generally understood the conditions of violence, impoverishment and services negotiation as individual pathology" (75–76). Terms like "low-income" and "client" worked to denote "an undeserving population of service recipients" (76). Client experiences were framed by service providers as being about problems with individuals' emotional states, not structural changes to the administration of programs (115). We can understand how clinical empathy, and larger practices within the medical humanities, would work here to reinforce for practitioners an emphasis on individual emotional coping while simultaneously diverting attention from structural inequalities. Delese Wear and her co-authors highlight a similar urgency in addressing the need for medical education to move away from the focus on individual empathy and toward social justice, most recently in relation to the tragic death of Freddie Gray and the systemic inequalities that his death brings to light (2017, 312–17). Wear et al. propose a change in medical curriculum that is "pedagogically oriented from two theoretical positions: antiracist pedagogy and structural competency" (313). The first provides opportunities for students to reflect on and understand the operation of power in their own lives; the second allows space for medical students to understand forces beyond patient–doctor interactions that affect health, from income inequality to decaying infrastructure and food deserts (313–14). With this kind of pedagogy, we can provide space for practitioners to recognize and interrogate the political economy of stigma within which HIV narratives circulate.

HIV Millennial and the Good Citizen

Most recently, HIV narratives have circulated with an attention to compliance and citizenship. This formulation of the good citizen is reinforced most recently by Paige Rawl, a young woman writing about her experience with HIV as an infant born with this condition. Rawl is the first "HIV Millennial" to write a book-length memoir; the memoir hit the market shortly after my reading groups ended.

What interests me about Rawl's memoir is how it functions as just one component of a larger package focused on public speaking and antibullying as seen on her website (http://www.paigerawl.com). Against a black background, we have a home page: on the left side is a red circle with Paige Rawl's name in cursive, with various descriptors of her underneath, including author, HIV/AIDS activist, and advocate against bullying. On the right side is a cover of *Scholastic* magazine, a midrange shot of Rawl, a young White woman with blonde hair smiling adoringly at the camera; the cover story is highlighted in yellow "Bullied by Her Best Friend." The cover of the memoir is on the right—a headshot of a young blonde woman with the title of the memoir in purple—*Positive*. The subtitle is in black cursive: "Surviving My Bullies, Finding Hope, and Changing the World." In teaching Rawl's book in my Disability Life Writing course, one of the things we talk about is her paratextual presence—everything that surrounds the book. This is clearly a book marketed within the young adult genre, and if you judge it based on its cover alone (and I encourage us to do so), we would never know that this is a memoir about HIV. Published in 2014, this memoir tells the story of Paige, born with HIV and raised by a single mother in Indiana. As Paige grows up and her HIV status is disclosed to her classmates, she becomes the object of bullying—not just by her best friend but by school officials. Eventually, she and her mother file an unsuccessful lawsuit, and she graduates and heads to college.

As readers, we are first introduced to Rawl by Jay Asher, a popular YA realistic fiction writer, who invites us readers to meet Rawl: "She will tell you in vivid, captivating detail her story—and it's a rollercoaster ride of emotion. It moves from heartbreaking to heartwarming, and will move *you* from feeling infuriated to uplifted to inspired" (v–vi). We have a male voice here telling us as readers exactly how to feel—and, of course, much has been written about disability life writing (and disabled representation more broadly) being used for inspiration porn, and I do think this introduction encourages that. But the inspiration is also framed within this idea that we are becoming "fast friends" with Rawl, which complicates this idea of objectification for the sake of inspiration.

Rawl introduces herself to readers in the preface, beginning with an image of seeing her own name scrawled with slander (which she does not repeat) on a public bathroom wall: "I never in a million years expected to see my name on this wall. I always considered myself to be a good girl—more Glee than Kardashians, more Taylor Swift than Miley Cyrus. I was born a joiner not a fighter" (xi). And this really begins the characterization of Rawl as an accidental activist, a good White girl whose HIV is as undeserving as the bullying. In framing herself this way, Rawl is speaking to the imagined White, middle-class female audience (young teens and mothers alike); she spends a lot of detail valorizing her own mother throughout the memoir (who contracted HIV through a husband who was cheating) and leading the readership to see her and her mother as an inseparable, misunderstood pair. Rarely do readers see the two engaging in HIV activism with others (there is one quick reference to their participation in a Pride parade in the early 2000s).

What is remarkable about Rawl's memoir is how she is able to completely ignore the question of sexuality—where most coming-of-age memoirs will address sexuality or a sexual experience, Rawl's memoir is surprisingly chaste. Never does she mention even conversations she might have with care providers about keeping herself and partners safe or other logistical questions that a young woman living with HIV would have in relation to sexuality. In claiming her White, good-girl identification, her book becomes about bullying: sexuality itself is the absent presence of the text. Rawl's memoir recreates deserving/undeserving divide within the HIV community that underscores Whiteness and heterosexuality, but it also does more than that: it obscures Rawl's HIV (the catalyst for the bullying by her peers and teachers) itself and frames the problem of living with HIV not as about lacking resources (educational, medical, etc) but as about people being mean. We can all understand Rawl's experience if we just have enough empathy. In fact, if the problem is not HIV but the social response to HIV—the stigma—then the cure for Rawl is itself empathy.

And, of course, this is a dangerous road to go down. I do not want to cite Rawl's memoir here in order to suggest there is a different or better way to tell her story—I want to cite Rawl's memoir to think about how what becomes legible shifts in relation to the political economy of stigma. When I have taught Rawl's memoir in Disability Life Writing courses with undergraduates, we often talk about Rawl's address to readers, the expectations of her audience, the frame within which she becomes legible. One student of mine, who identified as queer and disabled, found Rawl's framework repulsive and offensive; other students found it relatable, and others patronizing. And it can be all of these things at once because stories are never static, storytelling never simple. The political economy of stigma defines legibility as who can be an empathetic subject deserving of public support at a time when austerity reigns; it is who can be deserving of medical care when, as Puar explains in the time of Trump, "whose efforts to completely eliminate any whiff of socialized medicine are only really remarkable because they definitely expose the actual scale of disregard for human life, having blown so far open so quickly. Access to healthcare may well become the defining factor in one's relationship to the non-disabled/disabled dichotomy" (xvi). Disability life writing must be understood as a mechanism central to this health-care industry; those who do not have access to (appropriate) health care (because of the inability to frame themselves legibly on public assistance paperwork, because of an inability to frame themselves legibly to care providers) often do not in part because they are not telling the right story to the right people; the right story circulates and transforms alongside and within the larger political economy of stigma. When these narratives of disability are read differentially, through a differential consciousness, we can better understand how they unveil the production of debility and the clever ways in which readers debilitated within the political economy of stigma resist and transform that stigma, become uncontainable and unruly subjects.[1]

Narrative Medicine's Possibilities?

In part II, I critiqued the foundation of narrative medicine through founder Rita Charon's foundational 2008 text, her co-written 2017 text, my own participation in a weekend workshop, and its travels in another, pedagogical book with international circulation. Ultimately, I argued that narrative medicine as a brand fetishized narrative at the expense of patient privacy, doing nothing to address radical inequality—at times even perpetuating it. I want to turn now to one chapter in the 2017 co-written book, *The Principles and Practice of Narrative Medicine,* that provides a glimpse of possibility for addressing medical and social inequality; in doing so, I explore what it might look like for me to take a differential reading approach to narrative medicine.

In her only contribution to the co-written monograph, Sayantani Das-Gupta writes chapter 6, "The Politics of the Pedagogy: Cripping, Queering and Un-homing Health Humanities" (137–56). As I approached this chapter, I held my breath because I recognized concepts both foundational to my field ("cripping") and familiar to my politics ("queering"); I worried that these concepts would be appropriated, misunderstood, exploited. As I read, I let my breath out and began to feel connected.

DasGupta begins her chapter by expressly writing about how all pedagogy should be done with "a careful attention to power" (137), citing bell hooks, Chandra Talpade Mohanty, and Paulo Freire. Immediately I am transported back to the first semester of my PhD program and my feminist pedagogy class. DasGupta writes, "Hence, narrative medicine must insist on a hypervigilance against exploitation of inherent power of professional status" and asks, "Is it possible to search for such oppositional knowledge within the health humanities disciplines?" (138). Not only does DasGupta resist the branding of narrative medicine by using lowercase; she also insists on orienting her practice within larger fields with explicit histories and practices from marginalized communities. DasGupta locates herself as an able-bodied woman of color in relation to Sami Schalk's 2013 article, "Coming to Claim Crip" (cited in my introduction) (138).

---

1. I am inspired here by the work of Alexis Shotwell and Cynthia Barounis, both of whom write about notions of purity and citizenship and the political possibilities of, in Barounis's phrase, "antiprophylactic citizenship" (2–15).

DasGupta walks her readers through her journey as a professor of narrative medicine, looking back at her original 2001 syllabus for its absence of marginalized voices. She asks, in direct contrast to Spiegel and some of the other contributors to the book, "Who has access to language, the time to write, the ability to get published? Whose voices were we not hearing? I was compelled to ask these questions with my students time and again because of the overwhelming class, race and other privileges of the illness memoirists we were reading—there were few to no people of color, working class people, queer writers, and non-native English speakers in the bunch" (140). DasGupta cites how disability studies gave her the language to critique her own pedagogy, her own way of being "bound" to a medicalized lens (140). As her relationship to teaching narrative medicine became more complex, she writes of her recognition of needing to continuously challenge the doctor/patient binary. She writes that "cripping" her syllabus meant understanding her teaching as "an ever-expanding series of circles" addressing not specific diseases or conditions but "issues of body, voice, and self, caregiving practices, or embodiment and cultural identity" (142). She leaves her readers with an open-ended question: "Is it possible to truly incorporate a disability studies perspective and a medical perspective?" (143).

I want to tentatively answer DasGupta: perhaps.

Unfortunately, DasGupta was not one of the workshop leaders present when I participated in 2015. I wonder how my experience might have been different: Would I have been seen as difficult? Transgressive? Would the concept of ableism have been questioned as a term? More to the point now, what would it look like to take a differential reading approach to narrative medicine? I can only gesture toward this idea by suggesting a couple of observations, not meant to serve as a prescriptive "how to" but as one way to recognize my own conflicted positionality.

DasGupta, in a short essay for *The Lancet* in 2008, recognizes the trend of narrative entitlement (that I argue is produced by the political economy of stigma) within medical practice and proposes an alternative practice of narrative humility:

> Narrative humility acknowledges that our patients' stories are not objects that we can comprehend or master, but rather dynamic entities that we can approach and engage with, while simultaneously remaining open to their ambiguity and contradiction, and engaging in constant self-evaluation and self-critique about issues such as our own role in the story, our expectations of the story, our responsibilities to the story, and our identifications with

the story—how the story attracts or repels us because it reminds us of any number of personal stories. (981)

DasGupta's formulation of narrative humility is useful, adapted from the concept of cultural humility. It also recognizes that our identifications with a story, attraction or repulsion, are as much about our own experience as they are about the narrator's. What narrative humility does not do, however, is provide an analytic for narrative circulation, a way to understand trends in our own reception. Instead, for DasGupta, the practice of humility is the end point, the solution, to narrative entitlement, doing nothing to change, or even recognize, the larger power structures that enable narrative entitlement in the first place. Ultimately, our relationship to any text is mediated through a political economy of stigma—narrative medicine / Narrative Medicine indeed exists within this political economy, similarly to disability and illness memoirs themselves. Indeed, I do not believe that narrative medicine / Narrative Medicine would exist without the rising interest in life writing and the memoir boom at the intersection of an increasingly neoliberal health-care market. Narrative medicine itself is a product in circulation that unites the medical industrial complex with our increasingly neoliberal university system that values STEM fields over the humanities. In some ways, we can see narrative medicine as a clever way for humanities scholars to prove their utility in a neoliberal global market.

In July 2020 Sayantani DasGupta co-wrote with two narrative medicine colleagues a call for imagining abolition medicine in *The Lancet*. Here, Das-Gupta and colleagues call for a medicine that recognizes police brutality as a public health emergency and a continued recognition of how structural racism affects patient care amid both the COVID-19 pandemic and the ongoing police violence that led to the deaths of Breonna Taylor and George Floyd (158–59). I want to suggest that this abolition medicine can learn from the women living with HIV with whom I worked; a key component of abolition medicine can be differential reading. Differential reading means recognizing that all writing is shaped by structures of power. Differential reading means recognizing that all writing in book form is mediated through publishing genre expectations and paratextual circulation. Recognizing that this is different from the kind of reading between the lines that health humanities scholar Rebecca Garden suggests, writing, "All too often the person who is chronically ill or disabled is reduced to a stock role as a pitiable figure who serves to affirm others' normalcy and well-being, or as the 'good patient,' who must bear up stoically under the weight of suffering. By knowing how to read between the lines of these scripts and stock representations, clinicians can help their patients to resist them. By recognizing the ways that narrative conventions and social pressures can limit patients' stories of illness, clinicians can work with patients to renegotiate them" (2010, 122). Differential consciousness asks us not to read between the lines but to see the lines themselves as unstable. It asks us also to understand that narratives exist because the subjectivity of the teller has already been interpellated. There is no authentic story to find between the lines.

All writing is implicated in the structural powers at the intersection of oppression and privilege. By understanding power, and narrative itself, as a form of governmentality, we can understand that how a narrative meets or resists expectations is an exercise of the teller's negotiations of power. Recognizing this can mean the difference between using narrative for diagnosis and understanding narrative as part of a process of critical healing, what Garden defines as a practice that "resists reductive medical narratives by excavating the possibilities of meaning and by restoring the potential for multiplicities of story, particularly the narratives of bodily and psychic difference generated by those who seek healthcare" (2019, 1–2). Practices of differential reading also ask that we recognize a limited utility through finding connections between our own experiences and those represented by the narrative teller (patient/client/consumer/author). In the end, DasGupta's proposal of abolition medicine, if it includes a complex practice and understanding of differential reading, could begin to unravel, knot by knot, the political economy of stigma.

PANDEMIC POSTSCRIPT

I am currently completing my manuscript revisions during a surge of the worst global pandemic in 100 years. In the US, we have passed 500,000 deaths due to COVID-19, and that number is still increasing, even as we roll out a vaccine (Center for Disease Control and Prevention *Covid Data Tracker*; the *New York Times* "Corona Virus in the U.S. Latest Map and Case Count"). The last twelve months have left the American medical system under scrutiny, and while this book is critical of the medical system, I want to be clear that I am deeply grateful to first responders, particularly nurses and practitioners, who put their lives at risk to treat COVID-19 patients. Despite the best efforts of medical personnel, our current pandemic has highlighted significant failures in the current health-care system in the US. These failures can be understood, in part, through the political economy of stigma and the political economy of stigma can be better understood through these failures.

In an April 2020 article in the *New Yorker,* titled "What the Corona Virus Reveals about American Medicine," award-winning author and physician Siddhartha Mukherjee writes that we need to understand medicine itself as a "complex web of processes and systems" and that the pandemic itself has revealed fractures in this web (n. pag.). Many of us learned about the most publicized fractures—the failure to have a sufficient stockpile of personal protective equipment and ventilators this past winter and spring, the shortage of tests—what particularly interests me about Mukherjee's investigation is the way that medical providers were forced to exchange important clinical information in places like social media because of a lack of in-the-moment cohesive informational exchange network (n. pag.).

Mukharjee writes:

> That's because clinical medicine is, among other things, an information system, and a central part of that system is broken. Patient records that once were scribbled on clipboards now sit in electronic medical record (EMR) systems, many of them provided by the Wisconsin-based software company Epic. A standardized digital database of patient care records, searchable across hospital and medical care systems, could be an invaluable way of identifying effective approaches to a novel disease—like moving from a patchwork meteorological system where towns keep their own records of wind and rainfall to a national weather-tracking grid. (n. pag.)

As fellow physicians in the article discuss with Mukherjee the failures of the EMRs, they tell us that "almost all notes in the system are useless [. . .] Because notes are used to bill, determine level of service, and document it rather than their intended purpose, which was to convey our observations, assessment, and plan. Our important work has been co-opted by billing" (n. pag.). This is the technological environment in which patient narratives are being elicited.

I am thinking about this co-optation of EMRs at the same time that I am thinking about Professor Abigail Dumes's observations about evidence-based medicine. Her observations come in the context of an excellent anthropological investigation of the Lyme disease debates where she writes that evidence-based medicine, developed and institutionalized in the early 2000s and reinforced through the Affordable Care Act, does nothing to alleviate debates about truth in diagnosis and treatment. What evidence-based medicine does is open up questions for what counts as evidence itself—the distinction between signs and symptoms. For Dumes, this makes a huge difference in terms of what treatment gets supported by insurance infrastructures—the difference between those who believe chronic Lyme disease exists (the outsiders) and those who don't (mainstream medicine, insurance companies) (222–26). This in and of itself could be really interesting for the case of COVID-19 because we may find down the line a similar debate between acute COVID-19 illness (what we see and talk about now) and systemic or chronic COVID-19 illness—residual symptoms that could be treated and not cured, as in the case of Lyme disease. But what about evidence-based medicine, electronic medical records, narrative medicine, and COVID?

With the rise of evidence-based medicine, we have a platform offering a hierarchy of types of evidence, with objective evidence at the top and subjective at the bottom. Insurance and treatment protocols are based at the top of that hierarchy. Electronic medical records are created to document treatment for insurance standards—not holistic patient care. Therefore, the collection of narrative—the ultimate subjective reporting, both of patient and doctor—falls outside the parameters of American medicine.

I want to propose that medical narrative is becoming less relevant even as we have an increased interest in it; this opens up a place for an entirely new market through which to buy and sell patient narrative; but this new market, while outside of medicine, is actually intrinsic to it, similar to what Dumes writes about how mainstream medicine needs this system of evidence-based medicine where some bodies and symptoms are legitimized (and treated) and others fall outside. In Dumes's words, "Evidence-based medicine can be more fully understood as a technology of biopower [. . .] that simultaneously produces a categorical division between 'the right way to be sick' (medically explainable) and the 'wrong way to be sick'" (188). With the continuing rise of evidence-based medicine, with its placement of narrative as least important in the hierarchy of evidence, we can understand how and why electronic medical records fail to capture complex narrative experience. What the current COVID-19 pandemic has shown us is that this twinning of evidence-based medicine and electronic medical records creates a world where medical narratives exist outside the medical industrial complex, for the explicit purpose of legitimizing profit-based efficiency treatments. It is not an accident that medical narratives circulate within the political economy of stigma but is, actually, quite intentional.

APPENDIX A

Reading Group Bibliography

These are suggestions from which women in the group selected their top 4 or 5.

Black, Roxanne. *Unexpected Blessings: Stories of Hope and Healing*. Penguin, 2009.

Brown, Marvelyn. *The Naked Truth: Young, Beautiful, and (HIV) Positive*. Amistad, 2008.

Danquah, Meri Nana-Ama. *Willow Weep for Me: A Black Woman's Journey through Depression*. Random House, 1998.

Finger, Anne. *Past Due: A Story of Disability, Pregnancy, and Birth*. Seal Press, 1990.

Grealy, Lucy. *Autobiography of a Face*. Houghton Mifflin, 1994.

Hoffman, Regan. *I Have Something to Tell You*. Atria Books, 2009.

Hornbacher, Marya. *Madness: A Bipolar Life*. Houghton Mifflin, 2008.

———. *Wasted: A Memoir of Anorexia and Bulimia*. HarperCollins, 1998.

Lorde, Audre. *The Cancer Journals*. Aunt Lute Press, 1980.

Mairs, Nancy. *Waist-High in the World: A Life among the Non-disabled*. Beacon Press, 1996.

Peterson, Paula W. *Penitent, with Roses: An HIV + Mother Reflects*. U of New England P, 2001.

Sapphire. *Push*. Random House, 1996.

Slater, Lauren. *Love Works Like This: Moving from One Kind of Life to Another*. Random House, 2002.

Reading Group Discussion Guidelines

By participating in this discussion, I agree to:

Refer to women by their pseudonyms, for the sake of maintaining confidentiality.

Not refer to details that can be traced to a specific individual in the group outside of this discussion, for the sake of maintaining confidentiality.

Be respectful of others' experiences and beliefs.

Be conscious of body language and nonverbal responses—they can be as disrespectful as words.

Come prepared to discuss themes from the books, even if I read only a piece of that book.

Listen actively—respect others when they are talking.

Speak from my own experience instead of generalizing ("I" instead of "they," "we," and "you").

Not be afraid to respectfully challenge one another by asking questions but will refrain from personal attacks and instead focus on ideas.

Participate to the fullest of my ability—I want the group to hear my perspective!

Instead of invalidating somebody else's story with my own spin on her or his experience, I will share my own story and experience.

I have been informed that:

the goal of the group is not necessarily to agree—but to share our experiences.

Discussion Guidelines developed with the assistance of http://www.edchange.
org/multicultural/activities/groundrules.html.

WORKS CITED

Ahmed, Sara. *Living a Feminist Life*. Duke UP, 2017.

Banner, Olivia. *Communicative Biocapitalism: The Voice of the Patient in Digital Health and the Health Humanities*. U of Michigan P, 2017.

Banner, Olivia. "Introduction: For Impossible Demands." *Teaching Health Humanities*, edited by Olivia Banner et al., Oxford UP, 2019, pp. 1–15.

———. *Vulnerable Constitutions: Queerness, Disability and the Remaking of American Manhood*. Temple UP, 2019.

Basas, Carrie Griffin. "Private, Public or Compassionate: Animal Rights and Disability Rights Laws." *Earth, Animal and Disability Liberation: The Rise of the Eco-Ability Movement*, edited by Anthony J. Nocella II et al., Peter Lang, 2012, pp. 187–202.

Bell, Chris. "I'm Not the Man I Used to Be: Sex, HIV and Cultural 'Responsibility.'" *Sex and Disability*, edited by Robert McRuer and Anna Mollow, Duke UP, 2012, pp. 208–30.

Berger, Michele Tracy. *Workable Sisterhood: The Political Journey of Stigmatized Women with HIV/AIDS*. Princeton UP, 2010.

Berlant, Lauren. "Compassion (and Withholding)." *Compassion: The Culture and Politics of an Emotion*, edited by Lauren Berlant, Routledge, 2004, pp. 1–15.

———. "The Female Complaint." *Social Text* no. 19/20, Fall 1988, pp. 237–59.

Bersani, Leo. "Is the Rectum a Grave?" *October* vol. 43, Winter 1987, pp. 197–222.

Bérubé, Michael. *The Secret Life of Stories: From Don Quixote to Harry Potter, How Understanding Intellectual Disability Transforms the Way We Read*. New York UP, 2016.

Black, Roxanne. *Unexpected Blessings: Stories of Hope and Healing*. Penguin, 2009.

Bolaki, Stella. "Challenging Invisibility, Making Connections: Illness, Survival, and Black Struggles in Audre Lorde's Work." *Blackness and Disability: Critical Examinations and Cultural Interventions*, edited by C. M. Bell, LIT Verlag, 2011, pp. 47–74.

Brody, Howard. *The Future of Bioethics*. Oxford UP, 2009.

Brown, Marvelyn, with Courtney Martin. *The Naked Truth: Young, Beautiful, and (HIV) Positive.* HarperCollins, 2008.

Butler, Judith. *Giving an Account of Oneself.* Fordham UP, 2005.

Campbell, Fiona Kumari. *Contours of Ableism: The Production of Disability and Abledness*. Palgrave Macmillan, 2009.

Carter, Angela M. "Teaching with Trauma: Trigger Warnings, Feminism, and Disability Pedagogy." *Disability Studies Quarterly* vol. 35, no. 2, 2015.

Centers for Disease Control and Prevention. *30 Years of HIV in African American Communities: A Timeline*. n.d. https://www.cdc.gov/nchhstp/newsroom/docs/timeline-30years-hiv-african-american-community-508.pdf (accessed 2/18/18).

Centers for Disease Control and Prevention. *COVID Data Tracker*. https://covid.cdc.gov/covid-data-tracker/#cases_casesper100klast7days (accessed March 4, 2020).

Chambers, Ross. *Untimely Interventions: AIDS Writing, Testimonial, and the Rhetoric of Haunting*. U of Michigan P.

Charon, Rita. *Narrative Medicine: Honoring the Stories of Illness*. Oxford UP, 2008.

Charon, Rita et al. *The Principles and Practice of Narrative Medicine*. Oxford UP, 2017.

Clare, Eli. *Brilliant Imperfection: Grappling with Cure*. Duke UP, 2017.

Cleage, Pearl. *What Looks Like Crazy on an Ordinary Day . . .* Avon, 1997.

Cohen, Cathy J. *The Boundaries of Blackness: AIDS and the Breakdown of Black Politics*. U of Chicago P, 1999.

———. "Punks, Bulldaggers, and Welfare Queens: The Radical Potential of Queer Politics?" *GLQ: A Journal of Lesbian and Gay Studies* vol. 3, no. 4, 1997, pp. 437–65.

Colker, Ruth. *The Disability Pendulum: The First Decade of the Americans with Disability Act*. New York UP, 2005.

———. *When Is Separate Unequal?: A Disability Perspective*. Cambridge UP, 2009.

Couser, G. Thomas. "Disability, Life Narrative, and Representation." *The Disability Studies Reader,* edited by Lennard J. Davis, 2nd ed., Routledge, 2006, pp. 399–401.

———. *Signifying Bodies: Disability in Contemporary Life Writing*. U of Michigan P, 2009.

———. *Vulnerable Subjects: Ethic and Life Writing*. Cornell UP, 2004.

Crenshaw, Kimberlé. "Demarginalizing the Intersection of Race and Sex: A Black Feminist Critique of Antidiscrimination Doctrine, Feminist Theory and Antiracist Politics." *University of Chicago Legal Forum* vol. 1989, pp. 139–67.

DasGupta, Sayantani. "Narrative Humility." *The Lancet* vol. 371, 2008, pp 980–81.

———. "The Politics of the Pedagogy: Cripping, Queering and Un-homing Health Humanities". *The Principles and Practice of Narrative Medicine*. Eds Rita Charon et. al. Oxford UP, 2017, pp. 137–56.

DasGupta, Sayantani, and Marsha Hurst, eds. *Stories of Illness and Healing: Women Write Their Bodies*. Kent State UP, 2007.

Davis, Lennard J. "Constructing Normalcy: The Bell Curve, the Novel, and the Invention of the Disabled Body in the 19th Century." *The Disability Studies Reader,* edited by Lennard J. Davis, 2nd ed., Routledge, 2006, pp. 3–16.

Day, Ally. "Embodied Triumph and Political Mobilization: Reading Marvelyn Brown's *The Naked Truth: Young, Beautiful and (HIV) Positive.*" *Auto/Biography Studies* vol. 28, no. 1, 2013, pp. 112–25.

———. "Postfeminist Motherhood?: Reading a Differential Deployment of Identity in American Women's HIV Narratives." *Disabling Domesticity,* edited by Michael Rembis, Palgrave Macmillan, 2017, pp. 309–33.

———. "Toward a Feminist Reading of the Disability Memoir: The Critical Necessity for Intertextuality in Marya Hornbacher's *Wasted* and *Madness*" in *Disability Studies Quarterly,* 31:2. Columbus, OH. NP.

———. "Queering Boundaries of Body and Nation: Black Feminist Conceptualizations of Body in Illness Narratives." Unpublished MA thesis, Simmons College, 2007.

DeShazer, Mary K. *Mammographies: The Cultural Discourses of Breast Cancer Narratives.* U of Michigan P, 2015.

Diedrich, Lisa. *Indirect Action: Schizophrenia, Epilepsy, AIDS, and the Course of Health Activism.* U of Minnesota P, 2016.

Diedrich, Lisa. *Treatments: Language, Politics, and the Culture of Illness.* U of Minnesota P, 2007.

Dubriwny, Tasha N. *The Vulnerable Empowered Woman: Feminism, Postfeminism, and Women's Health.* Rutgers UP, 2013.

Duggan, Lisa. *The Twilight of Equality? Neoliberalism, Cultural Politics, and the Attack on Democracy.* Beacon, 2003.

Dumes, Abigail. *Divided Bodies: Lyme Disease, Contested Illness, and Evidence-Based Medicine.* U of Michigan P, 2020.

Edelman, Lee. *No Future: Queer Theory and the Death Drive.* Duke UP, 2004.

Eichorn, Lisa. "Applying the ADA to Mitigating Measures Cases: A Choice of Statutory Evils." *Arizona State Law Journal* vol. 31, 1999, pp. 1071–1120.

Elman, Julie Passanante. *Chronic Youth: Disability, Sexuality, and U.S. Media Cultures of Rehabilitation.* New York UP, 2014.

Erevelles, Nirmala. *Disability and Difference in Global Contexts: Enabling a Transformative Body Politic.* Palgrave Macmillan, 2011.

Feldblum, Chai R., Kevin Barry, and Emily A. Benfer. "The ADA Amendments Act of 2008." *Texas Journal on Civil Liberties & Civil Rights* vol. 13, 2008, pp. 187–240.

Foertsch, Jacqueline. *Enemies Within: The Cold War and the AIDS Crisis in Literature, Film, and Culture.* U of Illinois P, 2001.

Foucault, Michel. *History of Sexuality, Vol 1.* Translated by Robert Hurley. Random House, 1978.

Gagnon, Marilou, and Meryn Stuart. "Manufacturing Disability: HIV, Women, and the Construction of Difference." *Nursing Philosophy* vol. 10, no. 1, 2008, pp. 42–52.

Garden, Rebecca. "Critical Healing: Queering Diagnosis and Public Health through the Health Humanities." *Journal of the Medical Humanities* vol. 40, no. 1, Mar. 2019, pp. 1–5.

———. "The Problem with Empathy: Medicine and the Humanities." *New Literary History* vol. 38, no. 3, 2007, pp. 551–67.

———. "Telling Stories about Illness and Disability: The Limits and Lessons of Narrative." *Perspectives in Biology and Medicine* vol. 53, no. 1, 2010, pp. 121–35.

———. "Who Speaks for Whom? Health Humanities and the Ethics of Representation." *Medical Humanities* vol. 41, no. 2, 2015, pp. 77–80.

Goffman, Erving. "Selections from Stigma." *The Disability Studies Reader,* 2nd ed., edited by Lennard J. Davis, Routledge, 2006, pp. 131–40.

Gouge, Catherine. "'The Inconvenience of Meeting You': Rereading Non/Compliance, Enabling Care." *Feminist Rhetorical Science Studies: Human Bodies, Posthumanist Worlds,* edited by Amanda K. Booher and Julie Jung, Southern Illinois UP, 2018, pp. 114–40.

Gould, Deborah B. *Moving Politics: Emotion and ACT UP's Fight Against AIDS.* U of Chicago P, 2009.

Hammonds, Evelynn M. "Gendering the Epidemic: Feminism and the Epidemic of HIV/AIDS in the United States, 1981–1999." *Feminism in Twentieth-Century Science, Technology, and Medicine,* edited by Angela N. H. Creager et al., U of Chicago P, 2001, pp. 230–44.

———. "Seeing AIDS: Race, Gender, and Representation." *The Gender Politics of HIV/AIDS in Women: Perspectives on the Pandemic in the United States,* edited by Nancy Goldstein and Jennifer L. Manlowe, New York UP, 1997, pp. 113–26.

Hancock, Ange-Marie. *The Politics of Disgust: The Public Identity of the Welfare Queen.* New York UP, 2004.

Harrington, Anne. *The Cure Within: A History of Mind-Body Medicine.* Norton, 2008.

Harris, Cheryl. "Whiteness as Property." *Harvard Law Review* vol. 106, no. 8, June 1993, pp. 1707–91.

Hawkesworth, Mary. *Feminist Inquiry: From Political Conviction to Methodological Innovation.* Rutgers UP, 2006.

Hill Collins, Patricia. *Black Feminist Thought: Knowledge, Consciousness, and the Politics of Empowerment.* Routledge, 1990.

Hirschmann, Nancy J. "Freedom and (Dis)Ability in Early Modern Political Thought." *Recovering Disability in Early Modern England,* edited by Allison P. Hobsgood and David Houston Wood, The Ohio State UP, 2013, 167–86.

Hoffman, Regan. *I Have Something to Tell You.* Atria, 2009.

Holloway, Karla F. C. *Private Bodies / Public Texts: Race, Gender, and a Cultural Bioethics.* Duke UP, 2011.

hooks, bell. "The Oppositional Gaze: Black Female Spectators." *The Feminism and Visual Culture Reader,* edited by Amelia Jones, Routledge, 2003, pp. 94–105.

Iwai, Yoshiko et al. "Abolition Medicine." *The Lancet* vol. 396, no. 10245, 2020, pp. 158–59.

Johnson, Jenell. "Negotiating Autism in an Epidemic of Discourse." *Disability Studies Quarterly* vol. 33, no. 2, 2013.

Kafer, Alison. "Compulsory Bodies: Reflections on Heterosexuality and Able-Bodiedness." *Journal of Women's History* vol. 15, no. 3, 2003, pp. 77–89.

———. *Feminist Queer Crip.* Indiana UP, 2013.

Kannen, Victoria. "Identity Treason: Race, Disability, Queerness and the Ethics of (Post) Identity Practices." *Culture, Theory & Critique* vol. 39, no. 2, 2008, pp. 149–63.

Lejeune, Philippe. "The Autobiographical Pact." *On Autobiography.* Ed. John Paul Eakin. Trans Katherine Leary. Minneapolis: U of Minnesota Press, 1989, pp. 3–30.

Locke, John. *Two Treatises of Government.* Edited by Peter Laslett. Cambridge UP, 1960.

Marini, Maria Giulia. *Narrative Medicine: Bridging the Gap between Evidence-Based Care and Medical Humanities.* Springer International, 2016.

Martin, Emily. *Flexible Bodies: The Role of Immunity in American Culture from the Days of Polio to the Age of AIDS.* Beacon, 1994.

McRuer, Robert. *Crip Theory: Cultural Signs of Queerness and Disability.* New York UP, 2006.

———. *Crip Times: Disability, Globalization, Resistance.* New York UP, 2018.

McWhorter, Ladelle. *Racism and Sexual Oppression in Anglo-America: A Genealogy.* Indiana UP, 2009.

Metzl, Jonathan. *The Protest Psychosis: How Schizophrenia Became a Black Disease.* Beacon, 2009.

Mills, Charles W. *The Racial Contract.* Cornell UP, 1999.

Mintz, Susannah B. *Unruly Bodies: Life Writing by Women with Disabilities.* U of North Carolina P, 2007.

Mitchell, David T. "Body Solitaire: The Singular Subject of Disability Autobiography." *American Quarterly* vol. 52, no. 2, 2000, pp. 311–15.

Mitchell, David T., and Sharon L. Snyder. *The Biopolitics of Disability: Neoliberalism, Ablenationalism and Peripheral Embodiment.* U of Michigan P, 2015.

Mollow, Anna. "'When Black Women Go on Prozac': The Politics of Race, Gender and Emotional Distress in Meri Nana-Ama Danquah's *Willow Weep for Me.*" *The Disability Studies Reader,* edited by Lennard J. Davis, 2nd ed., Routledge, 2006, pp. 283–99.

Monette, Paul. *Borrowed Time: An AIDS Memoir.* Harcourt Brace Jovanovich, 1988.

Mukherjee, Siddhartha. "What the Coronavirus Reveals about American Medicine." *New Yorker,* 27 Apr. 2020. https://www.newyorker.com/magazine/2020/05/04/what-the-coronavirus-crisis-reveals-about-american-medicine. (accessed 11 Oct. 2020).

Muñoz, José. *Disidentifications: Queers of Color and the Performance of Politics.* U of Minnesota P, 1999.

Murphy, Michelle. *The Economization of Life.* Duke UP, 2017.

New York Times, The. "Corona Virus in the U.S. Latest Map and Case Count." https://www.nytimes.com/interactive/2020/us/coronavirus-us-cases.html (accessed March 4, 2020).

Nicolaidis, Christina. "What Can Physicians Learn from the Neurodiversity Movement?" *AMA Journal of Ethics* vol. 14, no. 6, 2012, pp. 503–10.

Nielsen, Emilia. *Disrupting Breast Cancer Narratives: Stories of Rage and Repair.* U of Toronto P, 2019.

Nielsen, Kim E. *A Disability History of the United States.* Beacon, 2012.

Nowak, Achim. "Disclosures." *Voices from the Edge: Narratives about the Americans with Disability Act,* edited by Ruth O'Brien and Rogers M. Smith, Oxford UP, 2004, pp. 55–69.

O'Daniel, Alyson. *Holding On: African American Women Surviving AIDS.* U of Nebraska P, 2016.

Pateman, Carole. *The Sexual Contact.* Stanford UP, 1988.

Patton, Cindy. *Last Served?: Gendering the HIV Pandemic.* Taylor & Francis, 2005.

———. "Women, Write, AIDS." *Gendered Epidemic: Representations of Women in the Age of AIDS,* edited by Nancy L. Roth and Kate Hogan, Routledge, 1998, pp. ix–xiiii.

People Living with HIV Stigma Index. *USA Michigan.* n.d. https://www.stigmaindex.org/country-report/usa-michigan/ (accessed 2/24/2021).

Peterson, Paula. *Penitent, with Roses: An HIV+ Mother Reflects.* Middlebury College P, 2001.

Pickens, Theri Alyce. "Pinning Down the Phantasmagorical: Discourse of Pain and the Rupture of Post-Humanism in Evelyne Accad's *The Wounded Breast* and Audre Lorde's *The Cancer Journals.*" *Blackness and Disability: Critical Examinations and Cultural Interventions,* edited by Christopher Bell, Forecaast 21, Michigan State UP, 2011, p. 75.

Pokempner, Jennifer, and Dorothy E. Roberts. "Poverty, Welfare Reform and the Meaning of Disability." *The Ohio State Law Journal* vol. 62, 2001, pp. 425–463.

Puar, Jasbir. *The Right to Maim: Debility, Capacity, Disability.* Duke UP, 2017.

Radway, Janice. *Reading the Romance: Women, Patriarchy, and Popular Literature.* U of North Carolina P, 1984.

Rak, Julie. *Boom! Manufacturing Memoir for the Popular Market.* Wiford Laurier UP, 2013.

Rawl, Paige. *Positive: Surviving My Bullies, Finding Hope, and Changing the World.* Harper-Collins, 2014.

Reach, Emily. "Invisible Illness and Incommunicable Diseases." TEDx Greenville, 1 May 2013, https://www.youtube.com/watch?v=VPWiCGSYtlw (accessed 4 Feb. 2018).

Roberts, Dorothy. *Killing the Black Body.* Vintage, 1998.

Russell, Marta. *Beyond Ramps: Disability at the End of the Social Contract.* Common Courage, 1998.

Samuels, Ellen. *Fantasies of Identification: Disability, Gender, Race.* New York UP, 2014.

——. "My Body, My Closet: Invisible Disability and the Limits of Coming-Out Discourse." *GLQ: A Journal of Lesbian and Gay Studies* vol. 9, no. 1, 2003, pp. 233–55.

Sandahl, Carrie. "Queering the Crip or Cripping the Queer?: Intersections of Queer and Crip Identities in Solo Autobiographical Performance." *GLQ: A Journal of Lesbian and Gay Studies* vol. 9, no. 1, 2003, pp. 25–56.

Sandoval, Chela. *Methodology of the Oppressed.* U of Minnesota P, 2000.

Sapphire. *Push.* Random House, 1996.

Schalk, Sami. "Coming to Claim Crip: Disidentification with/in Disability Studies." *Disability Studies Quarterly* vol. 33, no. 2, 2013, http://dsq-sds.org/article/view/3705/3240.

Scott, Joan W. "The Evidence of Experience." *Critical Inquiry* vol. 17, no. 4, 1991, pp. 773–97.

Scully, Jackie Leach. *Disability Bioethics: Moral Bodies, Moral Difference.* Rowman & Littlefield, 2008.

Segal, Jonathan A. "LEGAL TRENDS-Presumed Disability-Proposed EEOC Regulations Portend Vigorous Enforcement of the amended Americans with Disabilities Act," *HR Magazine* vol. 55, no. 5, 2010, pp. 95.

Siebers, Tobin. *Disability Theory.* U of Michigan P, 2008.

Simplican, Stacy Clifford. *The Capacity Contract: Intellectual Disability and the Question of Citizenship.* U of Minnesota P, 2015.

Shapiro, Johanna, Jack Coulehan, Delese Wear, and Martha Montello. "Medical Humanities and Their Discontents: Definitions, Critiques, and Implications." *Academic Medicine* vol. 84, no. 2, February 2009, pp. 192–98, https://doi.org/10.1097/ACM.0b013e3181938bca.

Shildrick, Margrit. *Leaky Bodies and Boundaries: Feminism, Postmodernism, and (Bio)ethics.* Routledge, 1997.

——. "Living On; Not Getting Better." *Feminist Review* vol. 111, no. 1, 2015, pp. 10–24.

Shotwell, Alexis. *Against Purity: Living Ethically in Compromised Times.* U of Minnesota P, 2016.

Smith, Robert J., and B. D. Agrawala. "HIV: The Invisible Epidemic of the United States Healthcare System." *Social Theory and Health* vol. 8, no. 1, 2010, pp. 83–94.

Smith, Sidonie, and Julia Watson. *Reading Autobiography: A Guide for Interpreting Life Narratives,* 2nd ed. Minneapolis: University of Minnesota. 2010.

Sontag, Susan. *Illness as Metaphor and AIDS and Its Metaphors.* Farrar, Straus and Giroux, 1990.

Spade, Dean. *Normal Life: Administrative Violence, Critical Trans Politics, and the Limits of the Law.* South End, 2011.

Spillers, Hortense. "Mama's Baby, Papa's Maybe: An American Grammar Book." *Diacritics* vol. 17, no. 2, 1987, pp. 64–81.

Spivak, Gayatri Chakravorty. "The Rani of Sirmur: An Essay in Reading the Archives." *History and Theory* vol. 24, no. 3, Oct. 1985, pp. 247–72.

Spivak, Gayatri Chakravorty. "Can the Subaltern Speak?" *Can the Subaltern Speak? Reflections on the History of an Idea,* edited by Rosalind C. Morris, Columbia UP, 1988, 2010, pp. 21–78.

Stone, Deborah. *The Disabled State.* Temple UP, 1984.

Sweeney, Megan. *Reading Is My Window: Books and the Art of Reading in Women's Prisons.* U of North Carolina P, 2010.

Titchkovsky, Tanya. "Absent Normalcy for Present Stigma: Goffman's Provocation." *Disability Studies Quarterly* vol. 34, no. 1, edited by Rosemarie Garland-Thomson and Jeffrey Brune, 2014, n. pag.

Tremain, Shelley. "Foucault, Governmentality, and Critical Disability Theory Today: A Genealogy of the Archive." *Foucault and the Government of Disability,* 2nd ed., edited by Shelley Tremain, U of Michigan P, 2017.

US Supreme Court. "Bragdon v. Abbott." *West's Supreme Court Reporter* vol. 118, 1998, pp. 2196–218.

Wald, Patricia. *Contagious: Cultures, Carriers, and Outbreak Narrative.* Duke UP, 2008.

Watkins-Hayes, Celeste. *Remaking a Life: How Women Living with HIV/AIDS Confront Inequality.* U of California P, 2019.

Wear, Delese. "The Colonization of the Medical Humanities: A Confessional Critique." *The Journal of the Medical Humanities* vol. 13, no. 4, 1992, pp. 199–209.

———. "The Medical Humanities: Toward a Renewed Praxis." *Bioethics Quarterly* vol. 30, no. 4, Dec. 2009, pp. 209–20.

Wear, Delese, and Joseph Zarconi. "Slow Medicine." *Gold Foundation News Room,* 15 Apr. 2015. https://www.gold-foundation.org/newsroom/blog/slow-medicine/ (accessed 3 July 2019).

Wear, Delese et al. "Remembering Freddie Gray: Medical Education for Social Justice." *Academic Medicine* vol. 92, no 3, 2017, pp. 312–17.

Wendell, Susan. "The Unhealthy Disabled: Treating Chronic Illnesses as Disabilities." "Feminism and Disability, Part 1," special issue, *Hypatia* vol. 16, no. 4, Fall 2001, pp. 18–33.

Williams, Patricia. "On Being the Object of Property." *Feminism: The Public and the Private,* edited by Joan Landes, Oxford UP, 1998, pp. 338–58.

Winnubst, Shannon. *Queering Freedom.* Indiana UP, 2006.

———. *Way Too Cool: Selling Out Race and Ethics.* Columbia UP, 2015.

Wooden, Shannon R. "Narrative Medicine in the Literature Classroom: Ethical Pedagogy and Mark Haddon's *The Curious Incident of the Dog in the Night-Time.*" *Literature and Medicine* vol. 29, no. 2, 2011, pp. 274–96.

Wyatt-Morley, Catherine. *AIDS Memoir: Journal of an HIV-Positive Mother.* Kumarian, 1997.

———. *My Life with AIDS: From Tragedy to Triumph.* Four Pillars Media Group, 2012.

Yagoda, Ben. *Memoir: A History.* Penguin, 2009.

Yergeau, Melanie. *Authoring Autism: On Rhetoric and Neurological Queerness.* Duke UP, 2018.

Young, Stella. "We're Not Here for Your Inspiration." *Ramp Up,* 2012. https://www.abc.net.au/rampup/articles/2012/07/02/3537035.htm (accessed 15 May 2016).

INDEX